Pediatric Intensive Care Nursing

Editor

MELISSA NUNN

CRITICAL CARE NURSING CLINICS OF NORTH AMERICA

www.ccnursing.theclinics.com

Consulting Editor
DEBORAH GARBEE

September 2023 • Volume 35 • Number 3

ELSEVIER

1600 John F. Kennedy Boulevard • Suite 1800 • Philadelphia, Pennsylvania, 19103-2899

http://www.theclinics.com

CRITICAL CARE NURSING CLINICS OF NORTH AMERICA Volume 35, Number 3
September 2023 ISSN 0899-5885, ISBN-13: 978-0-443-13099-1

Editor: Kerry Holland
Developmental Editor: Shivank Joshi

Critical Care Nursing Clinics of North America (ISSN 0899-5885) is published quarterly by Elsevier Inc., 360 Park Avenue South, New York, NY 10010-1710. Months of issue are March, June, September, and December. Business and Editorial Offices: 1600 John F. Kennedy Blvd., Suite 1800, Philadelphia, PA 19103-2899. Periodicals postage paid at New York, NY and additional mailing offices. Subscription prices are $160.00 per year for US individuals, $456.00 per year for US institutions, $100.00 per year for US students and residents, $206.00 per year for Canadian individuals, $573.00 per year for Canadian institutions, $230.00 per year for international individuals, $573.00 per year for international institutions, $115.00 per year for international students/residents and $100.00 per year for Canadian students/residents. To receive student/resident rate, orders must be accompanied by name of affiliated institution, data of term, and the *signature* of program/residency coordinator on institution letterhead. Orders will be billed at individual rate until proof of status is received. Foreign air speed delivery is included in all *Clinics* subscription prices. All prices are subject to change without notice. **POSTMASTER:** Send address changes to *Critical Care Nursing Clinics of North America*, Elsevier Health Sciences Division, Subscription Customer Service, 3251 Riverport Lane, Maryland Heights, MO 63043. **Customer Service: 1-800-654-2452 (US and Canada); 314-447-8871 (outside US and Canada). Fax: 314-447-8029. E-mail:** JournalsCustomerService-usa@elsevier.com **(for print support)** and JournalsOnlineSupport-usa@elsevier.com **(for online support).**

Reprints. For copies of 100 or more of articles in this publication, please contact the Commercial Reprints Department, Elsevier Inc., 360 Park Avenue South, New York, New York, 10010-1710; Tel.: 212-633-3874, Fax: 212-633-3820, and E-mail: reprints@elsevier.com.

Critical Care Nursing Clinics of North America is covered in *MEDLINE/PubMed (Index Medicus), International Nursing Index, Nursing Citation Index, Cumulative Index to Nursing and Allied Health Literature, and RNdex Top 100.*

Contributors

CONSULTING EDITOR

DEBORAH GARBEE, PhD, APRN, ACNS-BC, FCNS
Associate Dean for Professional Practice, Community Service and Advanced Nursing Practice, Professor of Clinical Nursing, Louisiana State University Health Sciences Center New Orleans School of Nursing, New Orleans, Louisiana

EDITOR

MELISSA NUNN, DNP, APRN, CPNP-PC/AC, CNE, NEA-BC
Instructor of Nursing, Louisiana State University Health, New Orleans, School of Nursing, Director of Advanced Practice, Children's Hospital New Orleans, New Orleans, Louisiana

AUTHORS

LEAH APALODIMAS, MSN, APN, CCRN, CPNP-AC/PC
Volunteer Instructor, College of Nursing, The University of Tennessee Health Science Center, Division of Pediatric Cardiology, Le Bonheur Children's Hospital, Memphis, Tennessee

LINDSEY BIRD, DNP, APN, CPNP-AC, CNE
Instructor, College of Nursing, The University of Tennessee Health Science Center, Division of Pediatric Cardiology, Le Bonheur Children's Hospital, Memphis, Tennessee

JACKIE CALHOUN, DNP, RN, CPNP-AC, CCRN
Pediatric Critical Care Nurse Practitioner, UPMC Children's Hospital of Pittsburgh, Assistant Professor, The University of Pittsburgh, School of Nursing, Wexford, Pennsylvania

BENITA N. CHATMON, PhD, MSN, RN, CNE
Assistant Dean for Clinical Nursing Education, Assistant Professor, Louisiana State University Health Sciences Center New Orleans School of Nursing, New Orleans, Louisiana

STEVIA DAVIS, MSN, PNP-PC, FNP
Pediatric Palliative Care, Children's Hospital of New Orleans, New Orleans, Louisiana

LAUREN K. FLAGG, DNP, APRN, CPNP-AC
Yale University School of Nursing, Yale New Haven Hospital Pediatric Critical Care, New Haven, Connecticut

HEATHER HERRERA, RN, MSN, CPNP-AC/PC
Christus Children's, San Antonio, Texas

CYNTHIA HOWES, MS, CPNP-AC
Pediatric Critical Care Nurse Practitioner, Department of Pediatric Critical Care, University of Maryland Children's Hospital, Baltimore, Maryland

VANESSA KALIS, DNP, CPNP-AC, ACNP, CNS, CHSE, FAANP
Division of Critical Care, Children's Hospital of Orange County, Orange, California

ALICIA KLEINHANS, DNP, MSN-Ed, APRN, CPNP-AC
University of Houston, Baylor College of Medicine, Houston, Texas

ANDREA KLINE-TILFORD, PhD, CPNP-AC/PC, FCCM, FAAN
Nurse Practitioner Director, University of Michigan Health System, Ann Arbor, Michigan

SARA T. LASS, DNP, APRN, CPNP-AC
Nurse Practitioner, Cardiac Intensive Care Unit, Children's Hospital New Orleans, Metairie, Louisiana

JENNIFER A. MAUNEY, DNP, APRN, CPNP-AC
University of Florida College of Nursing, Gainesville, Florida

BRIEANN MAURER, MSN, CPNP-AC
Pediatric Critical Care Nurse Practitioner, Department of Pediatric Critical Care, University of Maryland Children's Hospital, Baltimore, Maryland

EXIE MEREDITH, DNP, APRN, CPNP-AC
Baylor College of Medicine, Houston, Texas

JULIANNE MOSS, MS, CPNP-AC
Department of Pediatric Critical Care, Pediatric Critical Care Nurse Practitioner, University of Maryland Children's Hospital, Baltimore, Maryland

MELISSA NUNN, DNP, APRN, CPNP-PC/AC, CNE, NEA-BC
Instructor of Nursing, Louisiana State University Health, New Orleans, School of Nursing, Director of Advanced Practice, Children's Hospital New Orleans, New Orleans, Louisiana

DIANNE RICHOUX, MSN, RN, CPN
Assistant Professor of Nursing, Nicholls State University, School of Nursing, Thibodaux, Louisiana

DANIELLE SEBBENS, DNP, CPNP-AC/PC
Associate Director, DNP Program, Edson College of Nursing and Health Innovation, Arizona State University, Phoenix, Arizona

JESSICA L. SPRUIT, DNP, CPNP-AC, CPHON, BMTCN
Pediatric Nurse Practitioner, Stepping Stones Pediatric Palliative Care Program, Pediatric Blood and Marrow Transplant, C.S. Mott Children's Hospital, Ann Arbor, Michigan

BRITTANY SWEENEY, MSN, RN
Instructor of Nursing, Nicholls State University, School of Nursing, Thibodaux, Louisiana

JENILEA THOMAS, APRN, MSN, CPNP AC/PC, NNP
Texas Children's Hospital, Houston, Texas

JUDY VERGER, PhD, RN, CPNP-AC, FAAN
Adjunct Professor, College of Nursing, University of Iowa, Iowa City, Iowa

DANIELLE WOOD, DNP, CPNP-AC
Assistant Professor, Duke University Hospital, Durham, North Carolina

Contents

> Pediatric pain has historically been difficult to assess and even more diffi-
> cult to treat. It is encouraging that there is current research regarding pain
> control in pediatric patients that provide evidence for treating pediatric
> pain. Patients in a pediatric intensive care setting demonstrate a great
> deal of patient variability with regard to patient diagnosis, age, develop-
> mental level, weight, and amount of pain control needed. The use of an evi-
> dence-based protocol for pediatric pain control can decrease variability in
> pain control and decrease potential adverse effects such as respiratory
> depression, constipation, withdrawal, delirium, and developmental delays
> while allowing for patient variability.

> With supporting the best neurodevelopmental outcomes possible, the
> doctor of nursing practice project was constructed. An educational pro-
> gram was created for nursing staff discussing the importance of kangaroo
> care and how to safely facilitate it in the intensive care setting. Following
> the education completion, kangaroo care was implemented. Data were
> collected exploring barriers to implementation, discharge on maternal
> breast milk, and parental feedback.

> Pediatric critical care nursing is a key pillar in patient care and outcomes
> for children who are ill and injured. Tremendous advances have occurred
> in pediatric critical care and nursing. This article provides an overview of
> the key advances in pediatric critical care nursing through the decades.

> Health care providers caring for patients at the end of life (EOL) are faced
> with a multitude of emotions such as guilt, anger, sadness, and helpless-
> ness. Because of the negative impact of initiating EOL care (EOLC) to the
> pediatric population, organizations must be proactive in instituting educa-
> tion and resources on EOLC. They must also provide advanced skills to
> nurses who take care of patients at their EOL. Understanding the conse-
> quences of providing EOL care to patients in the pediatric intensive care
> unit allows for better allocation of resources and support services for
> nurses. This improves patient outcomes and nurse retention.

Communication is a central aspect of nursing care and is especially important when pertaining to progressive illnesses and end of life. This article reviews basic palliative care terminology and outlines a variety of communication frameworks from the "dos" to the "don'ts." These communication strategies are meant to be added to the nurse's "toolbox" so that nurses may use them in various scenarios. These communication tools are meant to help mitigate the stress and discomfort nurses often feel when using palliative communication or delivering bad news.

Unplanned extubations (UEs) are common, potentially avoidable complications of endotracheal intubation among pediatric patients. UE can be associated with adverse patient outcomes including increased length of stay, hospitalization cost, and cardiorespiratory decompensation. Inconsistency in the definition of UE has led to underreporting. Staff must be able to recognize and intervene appropriately when an UE occurs. Risk factors have been identified and quality improvement initiatives aimed at reducing UE have shown to be effective in reducing the incidence. The lack of consistent definition may lead to underreporting and may not lead to effective quality improvement initiatives.

Most children admitted to the pediatric intensive care unit with a new or reoccurring hematology or oncology diagnosis are at high risk for developing a hematologic or oncologic emergency. Although these children represent a low percentage of pediatric critical care admissions, their acuity is high, and their care is complicated and challenging. Nurses are an essential part of the interprofessional team of providers who care for these critically ill patients. Experience recognizing acute decompensation and excellent assessment and communication skills significantly improve patient outcomes.

Delirium is a fluctuating level of awareness based on a physiologic disease process. Within pediatrics, delirium affects approximately 30% of patients admitted to critical care units and is associated with increased mortality, morbidity, length of stay, and care costs. Multiple pediatric critical care societies recommend the implementation of screening practices using validated delirium tools. Delirium remains underrecognized because of suboptimal screening and protocol implementation in pediatric critical care units nationally and internationally. The mainstay of delirium prevention and management is nonpharmacologic, focusing on normalizing a patient's environment, sleep/wake cycles, nutritional status, and activity levels.

Pediatric intensive care units (PICUs) rely on interprofessional communication and collaboration to mitigate the risk for medical error. To operationalize these tenets, many PICUs use multidisciplinary bedside rounds as the foundation of their workflow. Bedside nurse participation in rounds is inconsistent, diminishing the return on team investment in patient safety. Given this dilemma, some institutions have shifted from provider-led to nurse-led rounds. Here, the authors explore the rationale, experiences, and outcomes of implementation of nurse-led rounds within 4 PICU service lines.

Asthma is a complex chronic disease characterized by inflammatory disorder causing airflow obstruction due to inflammation, bronchospasms, and mucus plugging. Children who fail to respond to initial first-line therapies often require hospitalization, and many with severe exacerbations and near-fatal asthma require admission to the pediatric intensive care unit (PICU). Nursing care of these PICU patients requires close monitoring and excellent assessment of their respiratory status. Administration of medications, such as albuterol, methylprednisolone, magnesium sulfate, and sedatives, is needed. Close communication with the care team is vital, including providers and respiratory therapy, to coordinate care and to communicate assessment findings.

Pediatric intensive care unit nurses can be exposed to hundreds of alarms per patient they care for each shift. The exposure to so many alarms can cause nurses to be desensitized to future alarms and thus increase the time to respond to alarms. This is one of the largest patient safety concerns within health care today. Steps should be taken to mitigate the number of alarms nurses experience so that they can properly respond to actionable alarms.

CRITICAL CARE NURSING CLINICS OF NORTH AMERICA

SERIES OF RELATED INTEREST

Nursing Clinics of North America http://www.nursing.theclinics.com

---

THE CLINICS ARE AVAILABLE ONLINE!
Access your subscription at:
www.theclinics.com

Preface

Pediatric Critical Care Nursing: Our Past, Present, and Future

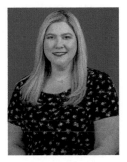

Melissa Nunn, DNP, APRN, CPNP-PC/AC, CNE, NEA-BC
Editor

Close to 250,000 children are admitted to pediatric intensive care units each year, and that number continues to rise as our care for this complex and vulnerable population improves. These units combine two specialties: caring for pediatric patients, which consists of understanding the child's developmental stage and ability, and working with their families, who are integral parts of their existence and critical care. As medical advances for pediatric patients continue, these patients are able to have increased life expectancies and greater quality of life. However, to achieve this, specialized nursing expertise has met and exceeded the challenge of providing such care.

Although nurses since the time of Florence Nightingale have recognized the need to stratify patients by acuity, the first critical care units began about a century ago in the 1930s. In order to understand the current state of pediatric critical care nursing, we need to understand our history, which will be addressed in this issue. It is hoped that recognizing our past will also inspire current pediatric critical care nurses, whether they are new to the profession or specialty or could write their own text on the advancements in intensive care nursing they have witnessed.

By examining our current challenges and successes, we can identify gaps in our collective research and practice that will enlighten the future of pediatric intensive care nursing. This will include acute pain management protocols, kangaroo care for neurodevelopment, comfort regarding providing end-of-life care, palliative care communication, preventing unplanned extubations, hematologic and oncologic emergencies, delirium screening, asthma care protocols, and battling alarm fatigue.

This issue of *Critical Care Nursing Clinics of North America* is dedicated to pediatric critical care topics that are frequently encountered when providing care for pediatric patients, including those experiencing exacerbations of complex conditions, those

Crit Care Nurs Clin N Am 35 (2023) xi–xii
https://doi.org/10.1016/j.cnc.2023.05.004
0899-5885/23/© 2023 Published by Elsevier Inc.

ccnursing.theclinics.com

with severe injuries, those undergoing complex surgical procedures, and patients and their families undergoing end-of-life planning and care.

Melissa Nunn, DNP, APRN, CPNP-PC/AC, CNE, NEA-BC
Louisiana State University Health
New Orleans, School of Nursing
Children's Hospital New Orleans
1900 Gravier Street, Room 330
New Orleans, LA 70112, USA

E-mail address:
mferni@lsuhsc.edu

Acute Pain Management Protocols in Pediatric Intensive Care Units

Alicia Kleinhans, DNP, MSN-Ed, APRN, CPNP-AC

KEYWORDS

- Pediatric - Acute pain - Evidence-based - Protocol

KEY POINTS

- Pediatric pain is difficult to assess and appropriately treat.
- Patients in a pediatric intensive care unit are highly variable.
- Use of evidence-based protocols can reduce adverse effects of pediatric pain control.

As many as 25% of all hospitalized pediatric patients experience acute pain and up to 70% of pediatric postoperative patients report moderate-to-severe pain.[1] Yet any exposure to pain can be detrimental to pediatric patients. Repeated or long-term exposure to pain can alter pain sensitivity or result in neuroanatomical abnormalities and emotional, behavioral, and learning disabilities.[2] Acute pain management in the pediatric intensive care unit (ICU) is an important aspect of care. Still, it can be inherently complicated with a narrow window of therapeutic management to provide adequate pain control while producing minimal adverse effects. Knowledge of pediatric pain management protocols may assist health-care providers because these evidence-based pain management protocols have been shown to decrease adverse effects, morbidity, mortality, ventilator days, and overall length of stay. This author attempts to describe the various categories of pain experiences of patients in a pediatric ICU, the evidence supporting the use of pain management protocols with pediatric patients and the assessment and treatment of the various types of pain using evidenced-based protocols.

BACKGROUND

Historically, pain in the pediatric population has been underrecognized and undertreated.[3,4] This has been attributed to many factors including mythology that children perceive pain differently,[5] difficulty of assessing pain in a nonverbal patient, parents being poor predictors of their children's pain[6–8] (Singer and colleagues, 2002, Chambers and

University of Houston and Baylor College of Medicine, 219 Marshall Street Apartment 117, Houston, TX 77006, USA
E-mail address: aliciakleinhans@gmail.com

Crit Care Nurs Clin N Am 35 (2023) 247–254
https://doi.org/10.1016/j.cnc.2023.05.001
0899-5885/23/© 2023 Elsevier Inc. All rights reserved.

colleagues, 1998 and Kelly, Powell and Williams, 2002), and concern for potential adverse effects when using opioids and benzodiazepines. There have been great improvements in knowledge of pain in the pediatric population. However, pain in neonates and infants is often excluded from studies due to the developmental differences in these ages. Additionally, pediatric patients with cognitive delays or disabilities may be excluded from studies due to the difficulty of adequately assessing their pain.[9] Improvements in adequately assessing pediatric pain and a greater understanding of the adverse effects of opioids and opioid dosing using adjunctive medications have laid the groundwork for the recent development of protocols for pain management in the PICU.

Acute Pain Management in Pediatric Intensive Care

Acute pain has been defined as pain with an abrupt onset that may be sharp or intense. Chronic pain is defined by Hockenberry, Rodgers, and Wilson[10] as pain that persists for more than 3 months. It is important for providers to not only target acute or chronic pain but to also consider that patients with chronic pain can have acute exacerbations while other patients may experience recurrent pain such as those with sickle cell pain, recurrent abdominal pain, and migraines.

Targeting different types of pain is not the only difficulty in managing pain in the pediatric ICU. There are many difficulties in creating a "one size fits all" protocol for pain management in a pediatric ICU setting. Patients in a pediatric ICU have various ages and developmental levels, which complicates assessing pain adequately. Children aged younger than 4 years are not able to self-report pain with typical pain scales. Additionally, the level of cognitive development may make it difficult to separate pain from emotion for many pediatric patients. There can also be a high variability of patient types. Many community hospitals do not have a pediatric ICU. Because these patients may be referred to a tertiary care hospital, the patients in a pediatric ICU can be a mix of patient ages and diagnoses or disorders. Many of these patients may experience acute pain due to surgical procedures. However, there may also be pediatric patients experiencing pain from burns, sickle cell crises, cancer treatment, and neurologic disorders. The combination of poor recognition of pediatric pain and the highly variable nature of patients within a pediatric ICU complicates the adequate management of pain.

Pain Assessment

Often the choice of pharmacologic management of pain is based on the patient's level of pain severity. Therefore, proper pain management in pediatric ICU patients begins with choosing an appropriate, validated tool for the population to assess pain levels adequately. The development and validation of tools to assess pediatric pain has dramatically improved the recognition and assessment of pain in pediatric patients. There are various types of assessments such as the self-report Wong-Baker FACES scale for children aged older than 4 years, behavioral scales for nonverbal patients including Face, Legs, Activity, Cry and Consolability scale, the COMFORT scale specifically developed for nonverbal patients in a pediatric ICU, and scales for neonatal patients including CRIES neonatal pain assessment scale and the premature infant pain profile.[11–13] A more in-depth examination of pediatric pain scales is beyond the scope of this article. However, pain management protocols for pediatric ICU patients should include and discuss the use of these validated tools.

Potential Adverse Effects of Pharmacologic Management

Controlling pain in pediatric ICU patients is not only humane but it can also allow a provider to perform procedures in an otherwise noncooperative patient, provide safety from dislodging arterial and central lines and endotracheal tubes, speed the healing time of patients and decrease potential long-term adverse effects. Some long-term effects studied include children experiencing PTSD from poor pain control during painful procedures.[5] Other long-term effects include altered pain sensitivity, neuroanatomical abnormalities, and emotional, behavioral, and learning disabilities.[2]

In addition to long-term adverse effects, short-term adverse effects, such as inadequate pain control, constipation, respiratory depression, withdrawal, delirium, mortality, or prolonged length of stay are important considerations. Some common medications used for managing acute pain include opioids and benzodiazepines. These medications are effective in producing analgesia, controlling pain, and controlling anxiety associated with pain and stimulation of the sympathetic nervous system. However, these medications also have a high potential for long-term and short-term adverse effects.

Opioids

The most reported adverse effects of opioid administration are vomiting, pruritis, and constipation. However, the most concerning adverse effect for patients receiving opioids is respiratory depression, which could lead to hypoxic ischemia or death.[14,15] Respiratory depression with opioid administration is of particular concern for patients with a natural airway, patients with a history of obstructive sleep apnea, obesity, prematurity, or developmental delay. A study by Fecho and colleagues[16] found opioids to be responsible for 50% of postoperative respiratory failure events. Other considerations for potential adverse effects of opioid administration are the large variability in patient responses, sometimes due to pharmacogenetics, and narrow therapeutic windows and withdrawal.[15]

Opioid dependence can manifest in as little as 5 days of administration of opioids. Physical dependence is a state of adaptation where a withdrawal syndrome can be seen when medications, particularly opioids, are abruptly decreased or discontinued.[17] A study by Ista and colleagues[18] found that withdrawal symptoms overlap with opioids and benzodiazepines. Due to the deleterious nature of withdrawal, controlled weaning of opioids and benzodiazepines should be included in a pain management protocol. An early study by Ducharme and colleagues[19] determined weaning rates for opioids and benzodiazepines to balance the reduction of adverse effects while avoiding withdrawal and can be helpful in protocol development.

Benzodiazepines

Initial studies encouraged the use of benzodiazepines as an adjunct to analgesia in pediatric patients, and it can still be seen in multimodal therapy for pain.[20] More recently, the use of benzodiazepines in pediatric ICU patients has been discouraged since findings of an association between benzodiazepine use and increased delirium in pediatric ICU patients leading to longer hospital stays.[21] According to Malas and colleagues,[22] the administration of opiates and benzodiazepines can double the risk for delirium. Delirium describes a syndrome of acute brain dysfunction that is extremely detrimental to patients increasing morbidity, mortality, and length of stay.[22] The study by Traub and colleagues[23] identified delirium as an independent risk factor of increased mortality in pediatric ICU patients. Due to these findings, judicious use of benzodiazepines in a multimodal approach to pediatric pain is recommended. However, according to a recent meta-analysis, benzodiazepines may still be used effectively as an adjunct to pain medication for procedural anxiolysis.[24]

Current Evidence

Current evidence in pediatric pain management has influenced pediatric pain management protocols and includes reduced usage of opioids and benzodiazepines, the use of adjunctive medications or a multimodal approach, and the study of pharmacogenetics. Reducing the use of opioids and benzodiazepines has been used by many providers given the risks of respiratory depression, withdrawal, and delirium as described above. A multimodal analgesic regimen using combinations of nonopioid analgesics may limit the need for opioids.[1,15] Adjunctive medications that do not have the adverse effect profile of opioids and benzodiazepines include dexmedetomidine, acetaminophen, and Nonsteroidal anti-inflammatory drugs (NSAIDs) such as ketorolac and ibuprofen.

Dexmedetomidine use has increased during the last decade with studies demonstrating it to be safe and effective in decreasing total amounts of opioids and benzo diazepines administered to children in a pediatric ICU.[25] Dexmedetomidine as an adjunct can potentiate opioid effects without additional respiratory depression.[15] Acetaminophen and NSAIDs have long been used for pain management because they have been shown to be safe and effective. Many providers have expressed concern over the risk of increased bleeding with the use of ketorolac. There are at least 2 well-designed studies that demonstrated no increased bleeding associated with ketorolac administration in pediatric postoperative patients. A prospective randomized trial of ketorolac after congenital heart surgery found no increased risk of bleeding.[26] After instituting a minimal opioid pain management protocol that includes ketorolac in pediatric cardiac postoperative patients, Frankel and colleagues[27] found no increased bleeding. Ketorolac can be a useful adjunctive medication in a pain management protocol in pediatric ICU.

The study of pharmacogenetics has rapidly increased during the past decade. Pharmacogenetics investigates the genetic variations in metabolism of medications.[15] Many opioids, including fentanyl, codeine, oxycodone, hydrocodone, tramadol, and methadone, are prodrugs, meaning they are converted to the active metabolite after entering the body. As described by Overholser and Foster[28] as well as Chidambaran, Sadhasivam, and Mahmoud,[15] these prodrugs are metabolized by enzymes in the CYP2D6 system. There are several genetic variabilities in CYP2D6 that result in some patients being poor metabolizers and others being ultrarapid metabolizers. Poor metabolizers may have a decreased response to medication administration, whereas ultrarapid metabolizers are at higher risk as excessive doses may be rapidly produced. Findings of pharmacogenetic studies have suggested that tramadol safety needs to be further investigated before widespread use due to reduced metabolic clearance with several medications. Additionally, ongoing studies on the safety of oxycodone regarding pharmacogenetics have been suggested.[15]

Development of Protocols

In caring for pediatric ICU patients, there is frequently considerable variation among providers for sedation and analgesia management.[2] With this high variability, there is a higher risk of poorly controlled pain and increased adverse effects including respiratory depression, withdrawal, and delirium. Managing interpatient variability in pain intensity and response to pain treatment while decreasing the risk of adverse reactions is accomplished with protocols.[1] Protocols have been shown to improve the morbidity and mortality of critically ill patients.[2,29] In a national survey by Rhoney and Murry,[30] the use of protocols for pain management in pediatric ICUs was very low in 2002. The authors hypothesized this was due to a lack of guidelines in the literature for pediatric ICU patients at the time.[30] They called for the development of protocols but progress took several years. Playfor and colleagues[31] developed one of the first protocols for pediatric patients based on Delphi technique (expert opinion) due to a paucity of evidence at the time.

Since this time, protocols have been developed for pediatric procedural pain, postoperative pain as well as pain and sedation protocols for intubated patients.[2,5,27] The following are examples of published protocols.

Procedural Pain Protocol

Crocker and colleagues[5] reported on a protocol for pain and anxiety in pediatric patients undergoing procedures in the Pediatric Emergency Department. Their protocol is divided into categories based on the patient's pain score. Interventions include nonpharmacologic measures for a pain score of 1 to 2, pharmacologic measures including acetaminophen and NSAIDs for a pain score of 3, and pharmacologic measures with a consult of a prescriber for a pain score of 4 to 7 as well as additional measures for a pain score of 8 or more. Medications in the category for pain score of 4 to 7 include oral hydrocodone/acetaminophen or acetaminophen/codeine or intranasal fentanyl, intravenous morphine or ketorolac for patients unable to take oral medications. If a patient reports a pain score of 8 or more, intravenous morphine is prescribed. This protocol is an example of multimodal analgesia for painful procedures, acute pain, chronic pain, or recurrent pain. An interesting finding of the implementation of the protocol was reduced remembered pain at discharge for both patients and parents.

Postoperative Pain Protocol

Frankel and colleagues[27] implemented a Minimal Opioid Postoperative Management Protocol for pediatric cardiac ICU patients. This protocol uses a multimodal approach with caudal anesthesia, dexmedetomidine, and scheduled acetaminophen and ketorolac. Opioids are prescribed per the protocol on a PRN or as needed basis. The addition of an opioid infusion may be added for patients on postoperative day 1 on a case-by-case basis as determined by the attending provider. Eighty-five percent of patients in this protocol were extubated in the operating room before arrival in pediatric cardiac intensive care unit (CICU) and an additional 3% were extubated within 8 hours.[27] Most patients received opioids postoperatively but opioid requirements decreased over time. In fact, 41% of patients received no opioids after day 1. The importance of this protocol is that it reduced the overall amount of opioids patients received yet maintained pain control with less than 10% of pediatric patients reporting more than mild pain.

Mechanically Ventilated Patient Pain and Sedation Protocol

Elella and colleagues[2] developed a pain management protocol that included the management of postoperative patients based on the expected time to extubation. Patients expected to be extubated within 12 hours were placed on a fentanyl infusion with acetaminophen and ibuprofen administration. A consideration of the addition of midazolam is outlined for patients expected to be extubated between 12 and 72 hours. Patients that remain intubated for greater than 72 hours have acetaminophen changed from scheduled to as needed with additional considerations to decrease withdrawal and delirium. Of note, this protocol was designed and studied outside of the United States. Findings from the use of this pain and sedation protocol included reduced ventilator days, ICU days, and overall reduced length of stay.[2]

DISCUSSION

Historically, pain in the pediatric population has been underrecognized and potentially undertreated, yet exposure to pain can be detrimental to patients. In pediatric patients, repeated exposure to pain can alter pain sensitivity and result in neuroanatomical abnormalities and emotional, behavioral, and learning disabilities. Some of the reasons for the underrecognition and undertreatment of pediatric pain were related to the mythology that children perceive pain differently, inadequate methods for measuring pain, and concern for potential adverse effects with medications typically used to treat pain and anxiety.

We know that children, including neonates, perceive pain and that perception of pain can be increased when considering the cognitive developmental level of the patient. There are now several validated tools that are helpful in assessing pain in a pediatric patient including self-report, behavioral, and tools specific for use with neonates. A validated tool for assessing pain should be part of any acute pain management protocol in a pediatric ICU.

Although there are serious adverse effects with the administration of opioids and benzodiazepines including respiratory depression, withdrawal, and delirium, they can be managed effectively with a multimodal approach. This multimodal approach can also address the large variability in patient responses, sometimes due to pharmacogenetics, and narrow therapeutic windows. The use of dexmedetomidine, acetaminophen, and NSAIDs such as ibuprofen and ketorolac allow for smaller overall dosing of opioids and benzodiazepines and are frequently utilized in current acute pain management protocols in pediatric ICUs.

Many protocols have been developed and found to be useful for procedural pain, postsurgical pain, and management of pain and sedation in mechanically ventilated patients. Some examples of recent protocols for these different patient scenarios have demonstrated reduced pain, reduced remembered pain, reduced use of opioids, reduced ventilator days, reduced ICU days, and decreased overall hospital length of stay.

SUMMARY

The use of evidence-based protocols for the management of pain and sedation in pediatric ICU patients can provide for adequate pain relief while decreasing the risk of adverse effects such as respiratory depression, withdrawal, and delirium.

CLINICS CARE POINTS

- Following an evidence-based protocol for acute pain management in pediatric ICU is beneficial for the patients.
- Using a validated pain assessment tool is vital to proper pain control in pediatric patients.
- Multimodal therapy with adjunctive medications such as dexmedetomidine, acetaminophen, and NSAIDs can reduce the overall exposure to opioids and benzodiazepines with minimal adverse effects.
- Monitoring patients for withdrawal is essential when weaning pain and sedation medications.
- Delirium has been found to be an independent risk factor for mortality and reduced exposure to opioids and more specifically benzodiazepines can reduce the incidence of delirium. All pediatric ICU patients should be monitored for delirium using a validated tool.

DISCLOSURE

The author did not receive any financial support for this report beyond the author's academic institutions. Furthermore, there are no personal financial interests or professional relationships related to the subject matter, and there are no patents or copyrights to disclose.

REFERENCES

1. Ferland CE, Vega E, Ingelmo PM. Acute pain management in children: challenges and recent improvements. Current Opinion in Anesthesiology 2018; 31(3):327–32.
2. Elella RA, Adalaty H, Koay YN, et al. The efficacy of the comfort score and pain management protocol in ventilated pediatric patients following cardiac surgery. International Journal of Pediatrics and Adolescent Medicine 2015;2(3–4):123–7. https://doi.org/10.1016/j.ijpam.2015.11.001.
3. Eland JM, Anderson JE. The experience of pain in children. Pain 1977;453–73.
4. Cummings EA, Reid GJ, Finley GA, et al. Prevalence and source of pain in pediatric inpatients. Pain 1996;68(1):25–31.
5. Crocker PJ, Higginbotham E, King BT, et al. Comprehensive pain management protocol reduces children's memory of pain at discharge from the pediatric. Am J Emerg Med 2012;30(6):861–71.
6. Singer AJ. Parents and practitioners are poor judges of young children's pain severity. Acad Emerg Med 2002;9(6):609–12. https://doi.org/10.1197/aemj.9.6.609.
7. Chambers CT, Reid GJ, Craig KD, et al. Agreement between child and parent reports of pain. Clin J Pain 1998;14(4):336–42. https://doi.org/10.1097/00002508-199812000-00011.
8. Kelly A, Powell C, Williams A. Parent visual analogue scale ratings of children's pain do not reliably reflect pain reported by child. Pediatr Emerg Care 2002; 18(3):159–62. https://doi.org/10.1097/00006565-200206000-00002.
9. Boric K, Boric M, Dosenovic S, et al. Authors' lack of awareness and use of core outcome set on postoperative pain in children is hindering comparative effectiveness research. J Comp Effect Res 2018;7(5):463–70.
10. Hockenberry, Rodgers, & Wilson. Mosby: (2022). Wong's Essentials of Pediatric Nursing, 11th Edition. ISBN: 9780323797580.
11. Crellin DJ, Harrison D, Santamaria N, et al. Systematic review of the Face, Legs, Activity, Cry and Consolability scale for assessing pain in infants and children: is it reliable, valid, and feasible for use? Pain 2015;156(11):2132–51.
12. Ambuel B, Hamlett KW, Marx CM, et al. Assessing distress in pediatric intensive care environments: the COMFORT scale. J Pediatr Psychol 1992;17(1):95–109.
13. Franck LS, Ridout D, Howard R, et al. A comparison of pain measures in newborn infants after cardiac surgery. PAIN® 2011;152(8):1758–65.
14. Jitpakdee T, Mandee S. Strategies for preventing side effects of systemic opioid in postoperative pediatric patients. Pediatric Anesthesia 2014;24(6):561–8.
15. Chidambaran V, Sadhasivam S, Mahmoud M. Codeine and opioid metabolism–implications and alternatives for pediatric pain management. Curr Opin Anaesthesiol 2017;30(3):349.
16. Fecho K, Jackson F, Smith F, et al. In-hospital resuscitation: opioids and other factors influencing survival. Therapeutics and clinical risk management 2009;5: 961–8. PubMed: 20057895.
17. Galinkin J, Koh JL, Committee on Drugs, Section on Anesthesiology and Pain Medicine, Frattarelli DA, et al. Recognition and management of iatrogenically induced opioid dependence and withdrawal in children. Pediatrics 2014; 133(1):152–5.

18. Ista E, van Dijk M, Gamel C, et al. Withdrawal symptoms in children after long-term administration of sedatives and/or analgesics: a literature review."Assessment remains troublesome". Intensive Care Med 2007;33:1396–406.
19. Ducharme C, Carnevale FA, Clermont MS, et al. A prospective study of adverse reactions to the weaning of opioids and benzodiazepines among critically ill children. Intensive Crit Care Nurs 2005;21(3):179–86.
20. Richtsmeier AJ, Barkin RL, Alexander M. Benzodiazepines for acute pain in children. J Pain Symptom Manag 1992;7(8):492–5.
21. Smith HA, Gangopadhyay M, Goben CM, et al. Delirium and benzodiazepines associated with prolonged ICU stay in critically ill infants and young children. Crit Care Med 2017;45(9):1427–35.
22. Malas N, Brahmbhatt K, McDermott C, et al. Pediatric delirium: evaluation, management, and special considerations. Curr Psychiatr Rep 2017;19:1–14.
23. Traube C, Silver G, Gerber LM, et al. Delirium and mortality in critically ill children: epidemiology and outcomes of pediatric delirium. Crit Care Med 2017;45(5):891–8.
24. Kuang H, Johnson JA, Mulqueen JM, et al. The efficacy of benzodiazepines as acute anxiolytics in children: a meta-analysis. Depress Anxiety 2017;34(10):888–96.
25. Czaja AS, Zimmerman JJ. The use of dexmedetomidine in critically ill children. Pediatr Crit Care Med 2009;10(3):381–6.
26. Gupta A, Daggett C, Drant S, et al. Prospective randomized trial of ketorolac after congenital heart surgery. Journal of cardiothoracic and vascular 2004.
27. Frankel WC, Maul TM, Chrysostomou C, et al. A minimal opioid postoperative management protocol in congenital cardiac surgery: safe and effective. Semin Thorac Cardiovasc Surg 2022;34(1):262–72.
28. Overholser BR, Foster DR. Opioid pharmacokinetic drug-drug interactions. Am J Manag Care 2011;17:S276–87.
29. Holcomb BW, Wheeler AP, Ely EW. New ways to reduce unnecessary variation and improve outcomes in the intensive care unit. Curr Opin Crit Care 2001;7(4):304–11.
30. Rhoney DH, Murry KR. National survey on the use of sedatives and neuromuscular blocking agents in the pediatric intensive care unit. Pediatr Crit Care Med 2002;3(2):129–33.
31. Playfor S, Jenkins I, Boyles C, et al, Neuromuscular Blockade Working Group. Consensus guidelines on sedation and analgesia in critically ill children. Intensive Care Med 2006;32:1125–36.

Implementation of Kangaroo Care in a Pediatric Cardiac Intensive Care Unit

Sara T. Lass, DNP, APRN, CPNP-AC[a],*,
Melissa Nunn, DNP, APRN, CPNP-PC/AC[b]

KEYWORDS

- Kangaroo care • Skin-to-skin • Congenital heart • Cardiac intensive care unit

KEY POINTS

- Newborns with complex congenital heart diagnoses requiring hospitalization struggle with neurodevelopmental milestones.
- Nursing facilitated kangaroo care between parent and newborn can help support neuro-development and overall outcomes.
- Main barriers to implementation of kangaroo care were the lack of parental presence and participation and nursing staffing shortages.

INTRODUCTION

Every year, about 400,000 infants worldwide are born with a complex congenital heart defect (CCHD) requiring some form of surgical intervention in the first months of life[1]. Although 85% of these infants are now surviving until adulthood, about half will be diagnosed with a neurodevelopmental disability.[1] These disabilities can include deficits in executive functioning, verbal skills, motor skills, and social cognition.[2] Studies have shown that abnormal sensory experiences in early infancy, such as hospitalization, may be the cause of these disabilities.[3]

The literature shows that kangaroo care (KC) in the initial phases of life can support brain development, decrease stress responses, increase parental bonding, and breast-feeding longevity.[4]

As such, a project was constructed to evaluate existing evidence regarding the use of KC in patients with CHD. This information was used to design a nurse training

[a] Cardiac Intensive Care Unit, Children's Hospital New Orleans, 1204 Elise Avenue, Metairie, LA 70003, USA; [b] Louisiana Health Science Center, New Orleans - School of Nursing, Primary Care and Acute Care Concentrations, Nursing Administration, 200 Henry Clay Avenue, New Orleans, LA 70118, USA
* Corresponding author. Cardiac Intensive Care Unit, 200 Henry Clay Avenue, New Orleans, LA 70118.
E-mail address: sara.lass@lcmchealth.org

Crit Care Nurs Clin N Am 35 (2023) 255–264
https://doi.org/10.1016/j.cnc.2023.05.002
0899-5885/23/© 2023 Elsevier Inc. All rights reserved.
ccnursing.theclinics.com

program and protocol to support infant neurodevelopment during hospitalization. Following education, this process was implemented as a new standard of care provided by nurses in the cardiac intensive care unit (CICU).

Background

Congenital heart malformations span a wide range of defects. More than 35 variations of heart defects exist, ranging from simple to critical.[5] The critical defects are typically life-threatening within the first days to weeks of life and require immediate intervention. Infants hospitalized within the first few weeks of life often require artificial airways, intravenous lines, multiple medications, feeding tubes, and monitoring equipment. Surgery may include cardiopulmonary bypass, the placement of additional intravenous lines and tubes, and require the patient to receive sedation and opioid pain control. While lifesaving, these interventions make it even more difficult for infants to adapt to their new environment outside of the womb. Sleeping patterns are interrupted, infant-parental bonding becomes a challenge, and the infant does not learn how to eat by mouth. Infants with CHD cannot leave the hospital until they can grow and gain weight. These connections are illustrated in a concept map (Appendix A).

Sleeping, eating, and bonding are crucial to the development of a newborn; they become the basis for physiologic and social development that extends throughout childhood. The developmental psychologist Erik Erikson identifies the newborn period as a critical time in the newborn's psychosocial development, in which a trust versus mistrust stage is established.[6] The parents' response to the infant's need for food, shelter, and comfort is necessary for the attainment of subsequent psychosocial developmental stages. Children who do not master this stage tend to struggle to feel safe and have difficulty attaining further psychological development.[6]

KC, also known as skin-to-skin care (SSC), is defined as: "when an infant is dressed in a diaper and held to a parent's bare chest," allowing for full skin-to-skin contact.[7] Research demonstrates that KC supports brain development, aids feeding, and increases physiologic stability. It also increases the frequency and length of time that mothers breastfeed.[8] Breastfeeding has been found to support maternal mental health while aiding in the infant's responses to infection and painful stimuli.[1] Even with the high level of evidence supporting its usage and cost-effectiveness, it was not used in the selected pediatric CICU.

Problem Statement

During clinical experiences, it became apparent that infants who spent extended periods in the CICU struggled with attaining expected developmental milestones in the hospital and after discharge. As documented by Erickson, one must master the first stage before moving on to subsequent development.[6] Although social work refers these infants to the early steps development program at discharge, not all patients will qualify for services. In addition, this program only supports these children for the first 36 months of life, and many of these disabilities can be lifelong. On consultation with those who specialize in these supportive therapies (physical therapy, occupational therapy, speech therapy), the question was raised; How could these children be better supported by bedside nursing throughout their treatment course in the CICU?

PICOT

The review of literature attempted to answer the following population, intervention, comparison, outcome, time (PICOT) question: Does implementation of a nurse-driven KC protocol result in an increased use of KC compared with patients who receive current care in the newborn population of the CICU over a 12-week period?

Available Knowledge

The information concerning the use of this intervention in this specific population was limited. However, there was high-level evidence supporting KC in infant development as an intervention overall. There were many studies concerning KC in the premature and low birth weight populations. Because research has shown that infants born with CHD have similar brain maturity to that of infants born at 34 to 35 weeks and both populations have similar neurodevelopmental outcomes, crossover of data is widely accepted.[9]

A systematic review of literature concerning neonatal-maternal separation investigated the importance of touch using skin-to-skin contact and its effect on stress regulation. This level of evidence would be considered Level 1.b according to the Joanna Briggs Institute (JBI) level of effectiveness. Articles that answered the research question were included if they contained empirical research that was peer reviewed, written in English, and published between 2015 and 2020. Articles that did not focus on KC or SSC for stress regulation and duplicate articles were discarded. Overall, the studies suggested that a decrease in heart rate variability should be considered a positive effect of SSC.[10] Maternal stress was significantly decreased when SSC was provided at least 3x/week. Infant salivary cortisol levels were significantly less in the SSC group after 60 minutes of skin-to-skin time ($P < .001$). Maternal and paternal oxytocin levels are increased, whereas cortisol levels are decreased following 30 minutes of SSC. SSC can regulate stress, anxiety, and psychological distress in both the infant and mother. SSC is considered safe in infants with a CCHD and has shown improvements in the infants' physiologic parameters. It was recommended that SSC should continue to be used as previously recommended by the World Health Organization even during a pandemic.[10,11]

A meta-analysis of kangaroo mother care (KMC) and neonatal outcomes was published in 2015 by the American Academy of Pediatrics in their official journal, *Pediatrics*. Randomized control trials and observational studies through April 2014 that discussed KMC and neonatal outcomes were included in the analysis. This would also be considered a JBI Level 1.b level of evidence. All gestational ages and birth weights were included. Studies with less than 10 participants, studies that did not have a comparison group, and studies without quantitative data were excluded. Synthesis of the studies showed KMC compared with conventional care was associated with a 36% lower mortality, decreased risk of neonatal sepsis, hypothermia, hypoglycemia, hospital readmission, and increased exclusive breastfeeding. Newborns receiving KMC had lower mean respiratory rates and pain measures. Higher oxygen saturations, temperatures, and increased head circumference growth were also observed. It is recommended that KMC should be used in all practice areas with newborns. However, practitioners should discuss strategies for KMC in reference to safety and feasibility per the specific care area.[4]

The Royal Children's Hospital (RCH) in Melbourne created a clinical practice guideline for KC in their CICU in 2020. The Nursing Clinical Effectiveness Committee reviews and publishes all guidelines for RCH. The guideline must pass the approval of the RCH quality and safety committee and it must be evidence-based and reevaluated every 3 years. Levels of evidence for the guideline include levels II–VII depending on the specific portion of the guideline addressed. Level II evidence is the highest in this case and it contains results from at least one large randomized control trial. The level II evidence in this guideline pertains to infants who receive SSC reaching full enteral feeds faster, having better thermoregulation, tissue oxygenation, neurobehavioral performance, and decreased need for pain medication.[12] Improvements in physiologic stability, sleep patterns, self-regulation, and weight gain, and decreased incidence of hospital-acquired infections (HAIs) were supported with lesser levels of III–VII. Caution must be considered in patients with lines and patients on respiratory support.[13]

Synthesis of Literature

The literature showed that KC is an important intervention for all infants. It should be used in all care areas for all newborns regardless of term age or birth weight. Newborns receiving KC had more physiologic stability (better vital signs, decreased pain responses), increased rates of breastfeeding, and decreased sepsis risk. Furthermore, infants receiving this intervention had decreased stress responses and cortisol levels. Parents are also noted to have decreased levels of stress hormones such as cortisol and increased levels of oxytocin which are seen in bonding and relationship building.

PROJECT DESIGN
Aim

The purpose of this project was to increase the use of KC in the CICU by 50% as a means of increasing maternal breast milk (BM) usage by 10%.

Outcome Measures

Goal 1: creation of an education session on KC with a content validity index (CVI) of at least 0.7. This was evidenced by averaging CVI data sheets from local experts. Goal 2: increase nurse knowledge of the benefits of KC by educating 90% of the nursing staff. Outcome was shown by attendance logs. Goal 3: increase the use of KC in the CICU by 50%. Outcome was measured by KC shift logs at each newborn's bedside. Goal 4: increase the use of maternal breast milk from 30% to 40%. Outcome measures were evaluated by Epic data search. The full project plan can be found in Appendix B.

The three key players in the success and function of the CICU were identified as: the unit medical director, the unit nursing manager, and the unit clerk. These were the three individuals noted to have the most influence on staff as well. The nursing manager role was filled by the interim who was active in creating the unit's practice guidelines. The medical director was noted to be invested in supporting this project, as there will likely be subsequent research opportunities initiated from its completion. The unit clerk was noted to have a large sphere of influence on the unit, especially with the bedside nursing staff. Also, the unit clerk was identified as the organizer of all records and documentation scanned into the electronic medical ecord (EMR). Initially, the bedside nursing staff was uninterested in being stakeholders for this project but was identified as crucial to its implementation and success. They were to be the individuals implementing the change and keeping track of progress on bedside logs. Other stakeholders included nursing education, ancillary therapies such as speech, occupational therapy (OT), physical therapy (PT), and integrative therapies. Although their multidisciplinary focus was important and may have been helpful in creating the initial KC education, they had low influence levels on the dedicated CICU staff. Parents were also identified as key stakeholders in providing KC. Without their buy-in, intervention does not exist.

Plan-Do-Study-Act Cycles

PDSA stands for plan, do, study, act. The PDSA framework consists of five design components: goals, content theory, education theory, data measurement and learning, and context.

Plan

This project's main goal was to develop a KC guideline specific to the CICU patient population based on current evidence-based practice. This guideline became part of a nursing education program discussing the importance of KC and how this intervention should be used in this care area. The education was constructed by the doctor of nursing practice (DNP) student using the evidence obtained in the review of literature. Educational content was reviewed by a cardiac intensivist, a neonatal nurse practitioner, and a certified healing touch practitioner for a content validity of at least 0.7.

The education program was disseminated via ELEMENO, a customizable digital educational platform, as an assignment for all CICU nurses. ELEMENO allows for training videos and lectures to be viewed using a user login on any computer and or smart phone through the downloaded application. Lectures were "assigned" as part of required ongoing nursing education to all nurses on the unit. Reports of how many views and which individuals have watched the lectures were generated with a 90% goal rate of participation.

The intervention targeted all newborns admitted to the CICU within the first month of life. Although the literature was not conclusive, the goal was to provide KC at least 3x per week between the infant and a parent for 60-to-120-minute sessions. Three sets of 4-week PDSA cycles were conducted. KC case logs were collected weekly.

Institutional review board (IRB) approval was submitted to LSU Health New Orleans before the initiation of the education. However, as the project was a quality improvement activity within the hospital, not generating new knowledge, and not generalizable to other settings, it did not require IRB oversight.

Do

Once staff completed the education, they were responsible for initiating the intervention and documenting it on a bedside log. Procedural guidance was provided by the KC unit protocol, also available at each eligible patient's bedside. The parents were also given a tip sheet on what to expect when providing care to their infant, which can be found in Appendix C. One log per newborn patient was used for each 12-hour shift. The log established if KC was able to be used and for how long. If the intervention could not be used in a shift, there was additional space to discuss what barriers occurred. Two logs (one for each shift) were distributed by the unit clerk or nurse tech every morning. The previous shift's logs were collected at the end of each week and stored in a central, secure location. These data were reviewed biweekly by the DNP student.

Study

The logs were reviewed, and the number of kangaroo sessions was divided by the total number of applicable patients. Once a patient meets 1 month of age, they were deemed to have aged out and the sessions were no longer counted. Data analysis of the KC intervention was then completed through a pre- and post-intervention t-test through SPSS to determine statistical significance of results. KC shift logs were periodically analyzed for noncompliance to assess barriers arising in real time. Reeducation and reevaluation of staff were addressed as needed throughout the PDSA cycles.

Act

From a cost–benefit analysis standpoint, KC has the potential to save the hospital thousands of dollars per year. The KC intervention itself is free of cost. The data showed that with the KC intervention, patients are more likely to exclusively breast-feed, potentially decreasing length of stay and increasing their resistance to HAIs[13]. A HAI requires 7 to 10 days of treatment with intravenous (IV) antibiotics. The cost of 24 hours in the ICU is approximately $1500. Medicare and Medicaid do not reimburse fully for HAIs, making it a costly expense for the hospital[6]. As such, this intervention should result in better patient outcomes, shorter lengths of stay, and decreased hospital costs.

Results

Over the 12-week period, five newborns were admitted to the CICU for management of their CHDs. Sixteen KC sessions were facilitated for two patients. The parents of these infants expressed high levels of satisfaction while holding and reported an increase in breast milk production. The two infants who participated in KC were discharged home on maternal breast milk.

Two patients did not complete any KC sessions due to parental refusal. In both cases, the DNP student was alerted to this barrier by the bedside logs. The DNP student then assessed the parent's understanding of the intervention and provided further education. One parent then held their infant four times, although not skin to skin, as there was concern for increased breast milk production, whereas the mother wished to formula feed. The family who refused KC altogether expressed discomfort related to too many lines/tubes and medical interventions that made them feel anxious to hold their child. Although the mother of the last newborn expressed interest in KC on admission, the patient was never hemodynamically stable enough for the physician and nursing team to feel comfortable facilitating holding sessions.

In reference to the four objectives stated at the beginning of the project, all were achieved.

Descriptive Analysis of Population's Demographics

Of the five total participants in the study four were females and one was male. Two were white, two were African American, and one was of Asian ethnicity. All were under the age of 30 days through the duration of the study. Data were no longer collected after 1 month of age per project criteria.

Analysis

During the first PDSA cycle, intervention implementation was low. Nurses had not completed assigned education, and providers were noted as a barrier. The providers in the CICU were uncomfortable that parents would be holding newborns with umbilical lines and lifesaving drips. Education had to be disseminated to the provider team to have them agree the benefits of KC were worth a potential risk. Comparative data were also obtained and presented to providers from the other unit that the KC guideline was adapted from to highlight the minimal risk of line/tube dislodgement. After this education, all providers, especially the advanced practice providers, became invested in providing KC to all eligible patients. Cycle 2 had the highest level of KC holding sessions. The goal levels of education completion were reached in this cycle. Unfortunately, during the last cycle, there were no more newborn admissions to evaluate.

Objective 1 was to complete education with a CVI of 0.7%. The CVI obtained was 1.0. Objective 2 was to increase staff knowledge of KC evidenced by a 90% completion rate of the assigned education in ELEMENO. A total of 27 out of 30 in the CICU completed the education resulting in a completion rate of exactly 90%. Objective 3 was to increase the use of KC as a bedside intervention from 0% to 50%. Out of the four eligible patients two completed care resulting in a 50% compliance rate. Objective 4 was to increase the use of maternal breast milk on discharge from 30% to 40%. Two patients were discharged on maternal breast milk, two were discharged on formula, and one remained inpatient, resulting in a rate of 50%. In reference to the PICOT question, although KC sessions were increased from a rate of 0% to 50%, the t-test resulted in a P value of 0.187 which speaks to insufficient evidence for statistical significance.

Observations

The two patients whose families refused KC were uninterested in breast feeding on admission. The mothers had already decided that they preferred to formula feed their infants.

Ethical Considerations

Although no correlation between refusal of KC and ethnic background can be drawn from this study, it poses the question of ethnic consideration. It is possible that there is a cultural component that may have been overlooked in reference to breastfeeding. Although there are data to support the positive benefits of breastfeeding, it may not be the accepted cultural norm in every household. The decision of whether to breast-feed an infant is culturally relevant and a sensitive topic for some families.

DISCUSSION
Strengths and Limitations

The biggest strength of this project was the dissemination of educational information. The platform ELEMENO made it accessible to all staff members involved. The limita-tion of this study was the sample size, and there was no way of anticipating how many newborns might be admitted to the center with CHD in the given 12-week period.

Sustainability

Since this study's conclusion, nursing staff has been facilitating subsequent KC ses-sions and more regular holding sessions with newborn patients. Education has impacted practice change, but the limitation of staffing shortages and safe patient ra-tios is still a challenge. The advanced practice providers have also proven to be advo-cates for providing KC to patients since this project's initiation.

Implications for Practice/Policy or Education

Practice change is ongoing and takes time and reinforcement, but this study initiated the process. The education and resources remain accessible to anyone who has an ELEMENO log in. All new graduate nurses will be assigned the presentation as part of their orientation to the CICU to create a standard of care. The KC guideline devel-opment is ongoing with the goal of eventually creating a unit policy.

Implications for Research

Further research is needed to identify ways to increase nursing compliance and parental comfort levels. There may be an opportunity to educate parents on what to expect in the CICU during fetal counseling visits for prenatally diagnosed CHD pa-tients. This could be an ideal time to discuss the benefits of maternal breast milk.

SUMMARY

Patients with CHDs are incredibly complex. Early hospitalization in the intensive care setting, while lifesaving, can cause significant delays in neurodevelopment. By imple-menting KC as a nursing-led intervention, better patient outcomes can be obtained. Although statistical significance in this study was not established, there was a notable change for the families involved. This type of impact, while verbally expressed by fam-ilies, is unquantifiable. The continued reinforcement of the importance of KC is needed to establish it as the standard of care in the CICU.

CLINICS CARE POINTS

- The early hospitalization of infants can provide abnormal sensory experiences and isolation from parents.
- Kangaroo care is a simple, cost-effective activity that can help negate some of these adverse effects on the infant and the parent.
- Safety must be prioritized as this population has a considerable risk of dislodgment of lifesaving lines and tubes.
- Parents should be educated on the benefits of providing kangaroo care and how to participate in this activity safely.
- Nursing staff should be educated and empowered to facilitate safe transfer of infants from cribs to parent's arms and monitor throughout the activity.

DISCLOSURE

The authors have no disclosures for this article.

REFERENCES

1. Harrison TM. Improving neurodevelopment in infants with complex congenital heart disease. Birth Defects Research 2019;111(15):1128–40.
2. Calderon J, Bellinger DC. Executive function deficits in congenital heart disease Why is intervention important? Cardiol Young 2015;25(7):1238–46.
3. Chorna O, Solomon JE, Slaughter JC, et al. Abnormal sensory reactivity in preterm infants during the first year correlates with adverse neurodevelopmental outcomes at 2 years of age. Arch Dis Child Fetal Neonatal Ed 2014;99(6). https://doi.org/10.1136/archdischild-2014-306486.
4. Boundy EO, Dastjerdi R, Spiegelman D, et al. Kangaroo mother care and neonatal outcomes: a meta-analysis. Pediatrics 2015;137(1).
5. Centers for Disease Control and Prevention. (2020, November 17). Critical Congenital Heart Defects. Centers for Disease Control and Prevention. https://www.cdc.gov/ncbddd/heartdefects/cchd-facts.html.
6. Cohen CC, Liu J, Cohen B, et al. Financial incentives to reduce hospital-acquired infections under alternative payment arrangements. Infect Control Hosp Epidemiol 2018;39(5):509–15.
7. Lisanti AJ, Buoni A, Steigerwalt M, et al. Kangaroo care for hospitalized infants with congenital heart disease. MCN: Am J Maternal Child Nursing 2020;45(3):163–8.
8. Zehra C, Rukiye T. The effect of early kangaroo care provided to term babies on the maternal-fetal attachment. Int J Caring Sci 2020;13(1):24–34.
9. Peterson JK. Supporting optimal neurodevelopmental outcomes in infants and children with congenital heart disease. Crit Care Nurse 2018;38(3):68–74.
10. Ionio C, Ciuffo G, Landoni M, et al. Parent–infant skin-to-skin contact and stress regulation: a systematic review of the literature. Internationalurnal of Environmental Research & Public Health 2021;18(9):4695.
11. World Health Organization. (2003). Kangaroo mother care a practical guide.
12. El-Farrash RA, Shinkar DM, Ragab DA, et al. Longer duration of kangaroo care improves neurobehavioral performance and feeding in preterm infants: a randomized controlled trial. Pediatr Res 2019;87(4):683–8.

13. Dam, E. (2020, January). The Royal Children's Hospital Melbourne. https://www.rch.org.au/rchcpg/hospital_clinical_guideline_index/Skin_to_skin_care_-for_the_newborn/.Guideline Purpose/Population: Clinical Nursing Guideline/Skin to skin care for the Newborn.

APPENDIX
Appendix A. Concept map

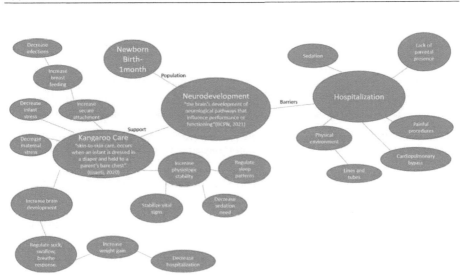

Appendix B. Project planning table

Objective 1	Creation of an educational session with content validity index of at least 0.7	Average CVI data sheets completed by 3 experts.
Objective 2	Increase nursing knowledge of the benefits of Kangaroo Care	Obtain 90% completion rate of assigned session in ELEMENO app.
Objective 3	Increase the use of KC as a bedside intervention from 0% to 50%.	Assess bedside KC shift logs weekly for compliance and barriers.
Objective 4	Increase the use of maternal breast milk from 30% to 40%.	Assess Epic data reports concerning discharge on breast milk.

Appendix C. Guideline and parental tip sheet

CICU Kangaroo Care Guideline

Population: Any newborn in the CICU from 0-1month of age.

Exclusions: Patients with an open chest, receiving ECMO, or on oscillator

Timing: Kangaroo care should be preformed 1-2x/day for 1hr sessions at least 3x/week.

Parent preparation: discuss timing of KC session with parent, advise them on the lines and tubes the infant has. Provide them with a hospital gown and blankets as needed. Ensure the call bell is easily accessible.

Infant preparation: infant should be dressed in only a diaper and hat. Confirm that alarm limits are set and appropriate for the infant's age.

Transfer: The bedside nurse should be available to orchestrate transfer of the infant to the parent's chest, and to the crib after care is completed.

Two nurses or a nurse and RT should assist with the transfer of an intubated patient.

Patient should be transferred to the parent's bare chest in a vertical position with arms and legs flexed, head turned to one side. Parent should have one hand supporting baby's head, one supporting their bottom.

Secure all lines and tubes to parent's clothing with enough slack for movement.

Wrap infant with parent's gown or a blanket.

During Care: the patient should be assessed every 30 mins during care. This responsibility can be shared with RT in a patient requiring respiratory support.

Infants who become unstable during care should be returned to their crib and the provider should be notified.

Encourage parents to speak to their infants, hum, or sing while providing care.

After care: assist parent in returning patient to their crib.

Secure all lines and tubes. Re-zero any pressure lines.

Document any instability in Epic as well as the provider notification and steps taken in resolving it.

Document the duration of the KC session on the bedside log.

Kangaroo Care Parent Tip Sheet

- Plan to spend at least 1 hour doing Kangaroo Care.
- Let your baby's nurses know when you will be coming so they can assist.
- Wear a loose-fitting shirt that buttons or zips in front. If you do not have this available a hospital gown can also be provided.
- Don't wear perfumes or smoke before providing care.
- Use the restroom and breast pump before starting.
- The nurse will assist you in transferring your infant onto your bare chest and covering them with a blanket. The nurse will also help in transferring your baby back to their crib when you are done.
- If your baby has a breathing tube the nurse or respiratory therapist must be called for all readjustments to keep your baby safe.
- Relax and enjoy the snuggles with your little one!

Evolution of Pediatric Critical Care Nursing

Jackie Calhoun, DNP, RN, CPNP-AC, CCRN[a],
Andrea Kline-Tilford, PhD, CPNP-AC/PC, FCCM[b],*,
Judy Verger, PhD, RN, CPNP-AC[c]

KEYWORDS

- PICU • Nursing • Pediatrics • Critical care • History

KEY POINTS

- Pediatric Critical Care continues to evolve.
- Nurses in pediatric critical care can transform outcomes.
- Interprofessional care delievery is optimal.

INTRODUCTION

Pediatric critical care (PCC) was recognized as its own specialty more than 40 years ago. During that time, independent children's hospitals with dedicated intensive care units were developed, and numerous advances in scientific understanding and medical technology were made. This article highlights the history of PCC nursing and its indispensability to the field of PCC, in addition to discussing many of the aforementioned advances.

1930S TO 1950S

Intensive care units (ICUs) were first developed in the 1930s to provide care for adults with poliomyelitis who developed respiratory failure and required treatment with "iron lung" ventilators. These units also cared for children with the disease. Around the same time, infants who had been born prematurely were being cared for in newly established units with specialized incubators, advances in nutritional support, and respiratory assistance, including the use of surfactant.[1]

Another development during this time period was the need for close postoperative monitoring of children who underwent increasingly complicated surgical procedures. General pediatric units were in existence, but it was becoming more clear that a different

[a] UPMC Children's Hospital of Pittsburgh, The University of Pittsburgh, School of Nursing, 3500 Victoria Street, 440 Victoria Building, Pittsburgh, PA 15261, USA; [b] University of Michigan Health System, Ann Arbor, MI, USA; [c] College of Nursing, University of Iowa, Iowa City, Iowa, USA
* Corresponding author. 656 Thayer Boulevard, Northville, MI 48167.
E-mail address: aklinetilford@gmail.com

Crit Care Nurs Clin N Am 35 (2023) 265–274
https://doi.org/10.1016/j.cnc.2023.04.001
0899-5885/23/© 2023 Elsevier Inc. All rights reserved.

type of unit was needed. The first dedicated postsurgical care unit in the United States was developed at the Children's Hospital of Philadelphia in 1956. Notably, this unit included a specialized team of nurses to care for these pediatric patients.[1]

Pediatric anesthesiology was the third important development during this time period. These practitioners bridged the divide between the operating room and the ICU and applied newly recognized differences in pediatric pharmacology and physiology to the care of their patients. Also, during this time, some pediatricians chose to receive additional education and training in anesthesiology to care for critically and acutely ill or injured pediatric patients.[1]

1960S

The first Pediatric ICUs (PICUs) were developed in the 1960s, when it was observed that critically ill children had improved outcomes when they were grouped together in the same unit.[2] At this time, all critically ill pediatric patients were cared for in the same unit, which included medical-surgical, neurological, trauma, and cardiovascular surgery patients, among others. These units combined the fields of pediatric surgery, pediatric cardiovascular surgery, pediatric anesthesiology, adult pulmonary medicine, and neonatology.[3]

Many of the first PICUs were established outside the United States. The first PCC unit was established in Sweden in 1961, followed by units in France and Australia in 1963, then in the United Kingdom by 1964.[3]

The first PICU in the United States was opened in the Children's Hospital of Philadelphia in 1967. The medical director of this unit was J.J. Downes, who was a pediatric anesthesiologist. This unit was followed closely by PICUs at Children's Hospital District of Columbia (1968) and at the Children's Hospital of Pittsburgh (1969).[4]

Care for children with congenital heart disease improved greatly during the 1960s. Surgical advances to repair these cardiac defects, such as the Blalock-Taussig shunt, were developed and implemented. The first balloon atrial septostomy was performed in 1968; this marked the beginning of less invasive pediatric cardiovascular procedures, which helped to improve the outcomes of patients with congenital heart disease while requiring less intensive postoperative recovery periods.[4]

1970S

PICUs continued to proliferate in the 1970s. Notable units included the PICU at Massachusetts General Hospital in 1971 and at Children's Medical Center in Dallas in 1975. Nearly all of the PICUs established during this time were within adult hospitals, as stand-alone children's hospitals were not yet commonplace.

The American Association of Critical Care Nurses (AACN) was established as the American Association of Cardiovascular Nurses in 1969 and by 1971 had transitioned to its current name. The AACN is a professional organization that provides support, education, and community for critical care nurses around the country. The Association held its first national teaching conference, the National Teaching Institute and Critical Care Exposition (NTI), in 1974. In 1976, the AACN developed its Critical Care Registered Nurse (CCRN) certification to recognize excellence and expertise in critical care nursing, including PCC.[5]

By the late 1970s, physicians were trained to become intensivists in PCC. This specialized training added further validation to the field and led to the opening of more PICUs across the United States and around the world.

Extracorporeal membrane oxygenation (ECMO) is a specially designed cardiopulmonary bypass that can be used to support cardiac and/or respiratory function over a potentially long period of time. In 1976, an infant with meconium aspiration was successfully treated with ECMO for the first time.[6] ECMO was also successfully used in pediatric cardiovascular patients. As with other developments in medical technology, the use of ECMO was facilitated by the burgeoning expertise of PCC nurses working in dedicated PICUs.

1980S

In 1982, the first Special Interest Groups were developed by the AACN. One of these groups was dedicated to PCC nursing. This group established a formal means for PCC nurses to collaborate, share their experiences and expertise, and grow their profession.[5]

The American Board of Pediatrics officially recognized critical care medicine as a specialty in 1985; this was the result of recommendations from the American Board of Anesthesiology, the American Board of Internal Medicine, the American Board of Pediatrics, the American Board of Surgery, and the American Board of Neurological Surgery. In addition to certification in general CCM, a physician can choose to further specialize in areas such as surgical, cardiovascular, or PCC with additional training and certification.[7]

Another major milestone in PCC medicine was the development of Pediatric Advanced Life Support (PALS) by the American Heart Association (AHA) in 1988. This development was preceded by a recommendation by the AHA in 1983 that a course for pediatric life support be developed. PALS teaches a systematic and organized method for the evaluation, management, and stabilization of injured and acutely ill pediatric patients, such as those experiencing respiratory failure or shock. The implementation of PALS improved the survival of these children from 10% to 85% over a relatively short amount of time.[8]

1990S

The 1990s saw the advent of several childhood immunizations that greatly reduced the incidence and severity of illnesses that once caused great pediatric morbidity and mortality. These vaccinations included those for *Haemophilus influenza type B* (HiB) (1990), hepatitis A (1995), varicella (1995), and *Streptococcus pneumoniae* (2000). For example, the varicella vaccine led to a 98% decrease in infection rates after its implementation; before the vaccine, an average of 4.4 million children per year contracted the disease, and many of these children required hospitalization. After the varicella vaccine, only 97,000 children per year contract the disease, and the severity of the illness is much lower. Another example of the success of childhood immunizations during this time period is the vaccine for HiB, which can be a cause of epiglottitis. This potentially fatal condition, which once required emergent tracheostomies and treatment with broad-spectrum intravenous antibiotics, was almost eliminated by the HiB vaccine.[9] In short, the childhood immunizations introduced in the 1990s dramatically changed the type and severity of disease with which children were admitted to PICUs around the country.

In 1999, the AACN introduced specialty certification for critical care clinical nurse specialists (CNSs).[5] This specialty certification recognized the experience and expertise of CNSs working in intensive care settings, including those in PICUs across the United States.

2000S

The certification for Pediatric Acute Care Nurse Practitioners (CPNP-ACs) was first offered by the Pediatric Nursing Certification Board in 2005.[10] CPNP-ACs were initially employed in ICUs, including both pediatric medical-surgical and cardiovascular surgery patients. Today, more than 4000 nurse practitioners are certified in pediatric acute care and work in a variety of settings, including intensive and acute care units, subspecialty clinics, and home-based settings.[11]

The American Association of Critical Care Nurse's Beacon Award was expanded to include pediatric units in 2008.[12] Award criteria recognize recipients based on excellence in leadership structures, staffing, staff engagement, communication, knowledge development, evidence-based practice measures, and outcomes.[12] The Beacon Award incorporates 3 tier designations on the journey to excellence and remains active today.[12]

This decade is also notable for the establishment and proliferation of multicenter research collaboratives in PCC. Some of the earliest formal research PCC collaboratives were established in this decade. The Pediatric Acute Lung Injury and Sepsis Investigators (PALISI), specializing in the prevention and therapeutic strategies for pediatric acute lung injury, sepsis, and other pulmonary and systemic inflammatory syndromes affecting children, was established in 2002.[13] Since its inception, PALISI has grown to more than 400 members.[13] Soon after, the Collaborative Pediatric Critical Care Research Network (CPCCRN) was founded (2004) to develop an infrastructure for well-designed collaborative clinical trials and descriptive studies to seek ways to reduce morbidity and mortality in pediatric critical illness.[14] The CPCCRN is funded through an arm of the National Institute of Health, specifically the Eunice Kennedy Shriver National Institute of Child Health and Human Development.[14] Since the launch of these PCC collaboratives, additional pediatric-focused research networks have been formed in many additional subspecialty areas. Research collaboratives provide a method to reach a larger enrollment for pediatric studies, with the goal to positively affect patient care. Pediatric ICU nurses are often integral in the work of these research collaboratives.

2010S

The concept of pediatric family-centered care gained support in nursing decades before its consistent adoption within the PCC sphere in the 2010s. This movement led to greater inclusion of families in areas of daily patient rounds, visiting, and decision-making.[15] The first guidelines for family centered care in neonatal, pediatric, and adult ICUs were published in 2017.[16] In addition, PICU architectural plans shifted toward the incorporation of single-patient rooms with designated "family space"; this often included pullout beds/sofas, miniature refrigerators, and workstations within PCC patient rooms.

The Society of Critical Care Medicine (SCCM) launched the ICU Design Award in 2013 to recognize an ICU integrating these physical features into new ICU spaces to promote attention to both functional and humanitarian issues.[17] The Ann & Robert H. Lurie Children's Hospital was the first recipient of this award.[18] The ICU Design Award remains active and is cosponsored by the Society of Critical Care Medicine, the American Association of Critical Care Nurses, and the American Institute of Architects Academy on Architecture for Health.[17]

Education through simulation saw significant growth during this decade, both high and low fidelity. This risk-free method of training expanded across many areas including resuscitation, procedural skills, clinical scenarios, and crisis management.[19–21] Use of simulation has been shown to be a powerful tool to increase performance, cognitive skill, and confidence while allowing opportunity to provide feedback and debriefing across health care disciplines.[19]

Sepsis, a leading cause of pediatric-health care utilization, morbidity, and mortality around the globe, received dedicated attention in this decade.[22] In 2002, with the partnership between the Society of Critical Care Medicine and the European Society of Intensive Care Medicine, the Surviving Sepsis Campaign (SSC) was born.[23] This joint initiative focused on reducing mortality from sepsis and septic shock worldwide through published evidence-based guidelines on early identification and management of sepsis and shock.[23] The establishment of published definitions for sepsis, severe sepsis, and septic shock was completed through collaboration at an international consensus conference.[22] The SSC, ongoing initiative with updated guidelines every 4 years, expanded its commitment to identifying the needs of patients through the lifespan by forming task forces specific to adults and children in 2016[22];this led to the publication of *Surviving Sepsis Campaign International Guidelines for the Management of Septic Shock and Sepsis-Associated Organ Dysfunction in Children* in 2020, a notable advancement in PCC for this decade.[22] PCC nurses are essential in the implementation of these guidelines through their role in advanced hemodynamic monitoring, pharmacologic therapy administration, nutritional support, and other advanced life-saving therapies.

Reduction of hospital-acquired conditions gained significant traction with PICU nurses as integral partners in progress on pressure injuries, ventilator-associated pneumonia, catheter-associated bloodstream infections, and indwelling catheter-associated infections.[24-28] Although much work was done by Curley and colleagues[29] (2003) to develop a pediatric pressure injury tool in the early 2000s, broad implementation of standard practice, benchmarking, and reimbursement implications lagged behind by more than a decade. Nurse-led care bundles to address hospital-acquired conditions are largely the responsibility of front-line nurses, often requiring adherence to documentation, checklists, and tracking.[30]

The 2010s also saw an increase in goal-directed therapy and nurse-led protocols to facilitate care and optimize outcomes in the PICU. Two areas of focus in this decade were extubation readiness and sedation titration. Use of an interprofessional team approach for creation and implementation of extubation readiness checklists became a prevalent strategy to promote successful extubation during this decade.[30,31] Nurse-led sedation protocols were developed and studied to promote algorithms to improve patient comfort and outcomes and reduce iatrogenic withdrawal.[32,33]

With improvements in care and survival for critically ill children over several decades, a new phenomenon was identified, postintensive care syndrome. This phenomenon was first described in adult patients surviving a critical illness and ICU stays and, subsequently, was extrapolated to pediatrics. This decade marked the development of the postintensive care syndrome in children (PICS-p) conceptual framework.[34] The PICS-p framework included multiple elements including the child's baseline status, psychosocial development, organ system maturity, and interdependence of the family at the time of critical illness.[34] The identification of PICS-p has resulted in the implementation of follow-up clinics to help reduce the impacts of the syndrome and maximize recovery.[35]

Similar to the advancement of technology and artificial intelligence in all aspects of life, these have also become critical tools in advancing care in the PICU. This decade was also notable for the implementation of pediatric scoring tools to recognize deterioration in patient status before it is overtly recognizable on physical examination. Earlier recognition of deterioration in patient status has led to earlier transfer to PICU care and improved patient outcomes.[36-38]

PRESENT DAY

Monitoring that was once available only through bedside monitors and central nursing stations has become more widely available on new platforms. Mobility and accessibility of patient data can lead to earlier identification of status changes and facilitate earlier adjustments to patient care. These tools are becoming more broadly accessible and with expanded interfaces with systems already adopted by hospital systems. New technology with more broad applications in this decade includes handheld/smartphone alarm notifications, streaming monitor data including waveform and heart rate monitoring, and enhanced communication for team members through secure text messaging.

The Coronavirus-2019 (COVD-19) pandemic resulted in infants and children being admitted to the PICU with acute disease and associated conditions. A new inflammatory process marked by a constellation of clinical and laboratory findings and COVID-19 infection was identified and defined as multisystem inflammatory syndrome in children (MIS-C) during the early phases of the pandemic.[39,40] Research quickly ensued to identify optimal management strategies for acute and critical children with MIS-C.[41,42]

The COVID-19 pandemic brought shifts in typical viral illness patterns, yielding more than a year of reduced hospital admissions for viral illnesses for respiratory syncytial virus (RSV), influenza, and other common pediatric viruses; this was quickly followed by an unseasonable increase in RSV infections starting in summer months of 2022 and a subsequent "tripledemic" of RSV, influenza, and COVID-19.[43] Relaxation of social distance and masking requirements in addition with inadequate vaccination rates accentuated the viral illness surge, requiring health systems and critical care units to devise plans to accommodate the surge in children with viral illnesses, straining an already strapped workforce.

Experiences through the 2020 COVID-19 pandemic yielded much sorrow and loss in personal lives, not only from patients and families but also from nurses and other health care workers. It pushed health care systems to rapidly shift care delivery models to incorporate more lean care delivery models, managing more patients with less staff. Multiple studies have highlighted the pandemic's effect on exacerbating long-standing burnout and exhaustion in critical care nurses including early departure from the profession.[44–46] In addition, moral distress, associated with challenges to professional integrity and lack of organizational support, was accentuated during the pandemic.[47] The widespread implications of burnout in health care workers has resulted in sounding the alarm and comprehensive recommendations by the US Surgeon General and National Academy of Medicine.[48,49] Further recognition that creating and sustaining healthy work environments with an embedded culture of psychological safety is imperative in combating burnout and moral distress to adequately support nurses' well-being.[47,50,51] Our patients and the health care system depend on the cultivation of a strong nursing workforce. This mission is critical in the current workforce landscape.

FUTURE

The future of PCC nursing is certain to bring ongoing advances in many facets of care delivery. Technology to enhance artificial intelligence in patient diagnosis and illness trajectory is likely to expand. Additional therapies are on the horizon, including an RSV vaccine that will change the landscape of PCC admissions and continued developments in personalized medicine. Further research in health care to promote equitable outcomes in PCC is essential to strengthening equitable and just health care delivery. Ongoing work to mitigate post-ICU syndrome in pediatrics to maximize outcomes while minimizing morbidities is essential to promoting healthy long-term outcomes for infants and children. A sustained commitment to a culture of caring is needed not only for patients and families but also for nursing staff and health care teams. And, dedicated strategies to attract and retain PCC will be essential to maintain the specialized workforce in this field.

SUMMARY

PCC has undergone significant transformations over the last several decades. This article has underscored many highlights of these advances and unanticipated changes, although addressing every change is beyond the scope of this article. Although technology advancements have shined, the commitment to providing patient and family centered care in an environment that promotes healing has significantly improved the experience for families in times of crisis and grief. Additional strategies are needed to support and heal PCC nurses and the health care team. The drive for sustained improvements in delivering safe, equitable, quality care continues to push innovation and advancements in PCC.

CLINICS CARE POINTS

- The first Pediatric Intensive Care Units were developed in the 1960s.
- Extracorporeal Membrane Oxygenation (ECMO) was first successfull used in an infant with meconium aspiration in 1976.
- The development of several childhood immunizations in the 1990s greatly reduced pediatric morbidity and mortality and admisssion to the PICU.
- Formal pediatric acute and critical care multi-center research collaboratives were established in the early 2000s, leading the way in improving pediatric critical care delivery.
- The 2010s were notable for earlier recognition of patient detrioration. * Coronovirus- 2019 (COVID-19) global pandemic was with a new particularly notable for inflammatory proecess identiftied as Muti-System Inflammatory Syndrome in Children (MIS-C) and widesweeping mental health impacts of on patients and heatlh care workers.
- The future of pediatric critical care will continue to expand technological and research advances in delivering safe, equitable quality care for children while focusing on the dedicated strategies to attract, maintain and support pediatric critical care nurses.

DISCLOSURE

None of the authors have financial interests to disclose.

REFERENCES

1. Epstein D, Brill JE. A history of pediatric critical care medicine. Pediatr Res 2005; 58(5):987–96.
2. Levin DL, Todres ID. Pediatric critical care. 4th edition. Maryland Heights, MO: Mosby Publishing; 2011.
3. Foglia DC, Milonovich LM. The evolution of pediatric critical care nursing: past, present, and future. Crit Care Nurs Clin 2011;23(2):239–53.
4. Levin DL, Downes JL, Todres ID. Review article: history of pediatric critical care medicine. J Pediatr Intensive Care 2013;2:2147–67.

5. American Association of Critical Care Nurses. History of AACN. 2023. Available at: https://www.aacn.org/About%20AACN/Complete%20History%20AACN. Accessed April 14, 2023.

6. Bartlett RH, Gazzaniga AB, Jeffries MR, et al. Extracorporeal membrane oxygenation (ECMO) cardiopulmonary support in infancy. Trans Am Soc Artif Intern Organs 1976;22:80–93.

7. Grenvik A. Subspecialty certification in critical care medicine by American specialty boards. Crit Care Med 1985;13(12):1001–3.

8. Bardella IJ. Pediatric advanced life support: a review of the AHA RECOMMENDATIONS. Am Fam Physician 1999,00(0).1743–57.

9. Talbird SE, Currico J, La EM, et al. Impact of routine childhood immunization in reducing vaccine-preventable diseases in the United States. Pediatrics 2022; 150(3). e2021056013.

10. Pediatric Nursing Certification Board. About Us. 2023. Available at: https://www.pncb.org/about. Accessed April 14, 2023.

11. Pediatric Nursing Certification Board. CPNP-AC Role. 2023. Available at: https://www.pncb.org/cpnp-ac-role. Accessed April 14, 2023.

12. American Association of Critical Care Nurses. Beacon Award. 2023. Available at: https://www.aacn.org/nursing-excellence/beacon-awards. Accessed April 14, 2023.

13. Pediatric Acute Lung Injury and Sepsis Investigators (PALISI). Available at: About Ushttps://www.palisi.org/about-us | PALISI Network. Accessed February 26, 2023.

14. Collaborative Pediatric Critical Care Research Network (CPCCRN).About Us | https://www.cpccrn.org/network-organization/about-the-network/CPCCRN. Accessed February 26, 2023.

15. Butler A, Copnell B, Willetts G. Family-centred care in the paediatric intensive care unit: an integrative review of the literature. J Clin Nurs 2014;23(15–16): 2086–99.

16. Davidson JE, Aslakson RA, Long AC, et al. Guidelines for family-centered care in the neonatal, pediatric, and adult ICU. Crit Care Med 2017;45(1):103–28.

17. Society of Critical Care Medicine. Awards. Available at: https://www.sccm.org/Member-Center/Professional-Development/Awards. Accessed April 14, 2023.

18. Society of Critical Care Medicine. Personal communication 2023.

19. Lin Y, Cheng A. The role of simulation in teaching pediatric resuscitation: current perspectives. Adv Med Educ Pract 2015;6:239–48.

20. Eppich WJ, Adler MD, McGaghie WC. Emergency and critical care pediatrics: use of medical simulation for training in acute pediatric emergencies. Curr Opin Pediatr 2006;18(3):266–71.

21. Youngblood AQ, Zinkan JL, Tofil NM, et al. Multidisciplinary simulation in pediatric critical care: the death of a child. Crit Care Nurse 2012;32(3):55–61.

22. Weiss SL, Peter MJ, Alhazzani W, et al. Surviving sepsis Campaign international guidelines for the management of septic shock and sepsis-associated organ dysfunction in children. Pediatr Crit Care Med 2020;21(2):E52–106.

23. Society of Critical Care Medicine. Surviving Sepsis Campaign Surviving Sepsis Campaign (SSC) | SCCM.

24. Cummins KA, Watters R, Leming-Lee T'. Reducing pressure injuries in the pediatric intensive care unit. Nurs Clin North Am 2019;54(1):127–40.

25. Cooper VB, Haut C. Preventing ventilator-associated pneumonia in children: an evidence-based protocol. Crit Care Nurse 2013;33(3):21–9.

26. Snyder MD, Priestley MA, Weiss M, et al. Preventing catheter-associated urinary tract infections in the pediatric intensive care unit. Crit Care Nurse 2020;40(1): e12–7.
27. Ullman AJ, Long DA, Rickard CM. Prevention of central venous catheter infections: a survey of paediatric ICU nurses' knowledge and practice. Nurse Educ Today 2014;34(2):202–7.
28. Sohail Ahmed S, McCaskey MS, Bringman S, et al. Catheter-associated bloodstream infection in the pediatric intensive care unit: a multidisciplinary approach. Pediatr Crit Care Med 2012;13(2):e69–72.
29. Curley MAQ, Razmus IE, Roberts KE, et al. Predicting pressure ulcer risk in pediatric patients: the Braden Q score. Nurse Res 2003;51(1):22–33.
30. Waak M, Harnischfeger J, Ferguson A, et al. Every child, every day, back to play: the PICUstars protocol - implementation of a nurse-led PICU liberation program. BMC Pediatr 2022;22:279.
31. Bankhead S, Chong K, Kamai S. Preventing extubation failures in a pediatric intensive care unit. Nurs Clin 2014;49:321–8.
32. Curley MAQ, Gedeit RG, Dodson B, et al. Methods in the design and implementation of the randomized evaluation of sedation titration for respiratory failure (*RESTORE*) clinical trial. Trials 2018;19:687.
33. Lincoln PA, Whelan K, Hartwell LP, et al. Nurse-implemented goal-directed strategy to improve pain and sedation management in a pediatric cardiac ICU. Pediatr Crit Care Med 2020;21(12):1064–70.
34. Manning JC, Pinto NP, Rennick JE, et al. Conceptualizing post intensive care syndrome in children-the PICS-p framework. Pediatr Crit Care Med 2018;19(4): 298–300.
35. Hartman ME, Williams CN, Hall TA, et al. Post-intensive-care syndrome for the pediatric neurologist. Pediatr Neurol 2020;108:47–53.
36. Skaletzky SM, Raszynski A, Totapally BR. Validation of a modified pediatric early warning system score: a retrospective case–control study. Clin Pediatr 2012; 51(5):431–5.
37. Akre M, Finkelstein M, Erickson M, et al. Sensitivity of the pediatric early warning score to identify patient deterioration. Pediatrics 2010;125(4):e763–9.
38. Lambert V, Matthews A, MacDonell R, et al. Paediatric early warning systems for detecting and responding to clinical deterioration in children: a systematic review. BMJ Open 2017;7:e014497.
39. Green J. Developing nursing knowledge on COVID-19 in children and adolescents: an integrative review. Pediatr Nurs 2021;47(4):163–74.
40. MaGowan N. Navigating through the uncharted territory of Multisystem Inflammatory Syndrome in Children (MIS-C): what the pediatric clinical nurse must know. Pediatr Nurs 2020;46(6):273–7.
41. Hennon TR, Penque MD, Abdul-Aziz R, et al. COVID-19 associated multisystem inflammatory syndrome in children (MIS-C) guidelines; a Western New York approach. Prog Pediatr Cardiol 2020;57:101232.
42. Algarni AS, Alamri NM, Khayat NZ, et al. Clinical practice guidelines in multisystem inflammatory syndrome (MIS-C) related to COVID-19: a critical review and recommendations. World Journal of Pediatrics 2022;18(2):83–90.
43. Tanne JH. US faces triple epidemic of flu, RSV, and covid. BMJ 2022;379:o2681.
44. Kissel KA, Filipek C, Jenkins J. Impact of the COVID-19 pandemic on nurses working in intensive care units: a scoping review. Crit Care Nurse 2023;1–20. https://doi.org/10.4037/ccn2023196.

45. Barr P. Dimensions of the burnout measure: relationships with shame- and guilt-proneness in neonatal intensive care unit nurses. Aust Crit Care 2022;35(2): 174–80.
46. Matsuishi Y, Mathis BJ, Masuzawa Y, et al. Severity and prevalence of burnout syndrome in paediatric intensive care nurses: a systematic review. Intensive Crit Care Nurs 2021;67:103082.
47. Thomas TA, Davis FD, Kumar S, et al. Rushton; COVID-19 and moral distress: a pediatric critical care survey. Am J Crit Care 2021;30(6):e80–98.
48. U.S. Department of Health and Human Services. Addressing health worker burnout: the U.S. Surgeon General's Advisory of Building a Thriving Health Workforce. Available: https://www.hhs.gov/surgeongeneral/priorities/health-worker-burnout/index.html. Accessed March 3, 2023.
49. National Academy of Medicine. National plan for health workforce wellbeing. Available at: https://nam.edu/initiatives/clinician-resilience-and-well-being/national-plan-for-health-workforce-well-being/. Accessed March 3, 2023.
50. Blake, Future of Nursing 2020-2030: supporting the health and well-being of nurses. AACN Adv Crit Care 2022;33(1):99–102.
51. Munro CL, Hope AA. Improving nurse well-being: the need is urgent and the time is now. Am J Crit Care 2022;31(1):4–6.

The Impact of End-of-Life Care Among Nurses Working in the Pediatric Intensive Care Unit

Benita N. Chatmon, PhD, MSN, RN, CNE[a,*],
Dianne Richoux, MSN, RN, CPN[b], Brittany Sweeney, MSN, RN[b]

KEYWORDS

- Pediatric intensive care unit • End-of-life care • Palliative care • Pediatric nurses
- Compassion fatigue • Moral distress • Job satisfaction • Burnout

KEY POINTS

- One of the most difficult aspects of pediatric nursing is coping with the death of a child.
- Evidence has shown that nurses do not have formal education or training in end-of-life care (EOLC), leading to barriers such as moral distress, compassion fatigue, burnout, job dissatisfaction, and decreased resiliency.
- Because of the negative impact of initiating EOLC to the pediatric population, organizations must be proactive in instituting education on EOLC and providing advanced skills to nurses who take care of patients at their EOL.
- The integration of EOLC curriculum into schools of nursing is highly regarded as a first step.
- Effective organizational support includes work engagement strategies, open and receptive communication, and educational resources.

INTRODUCTION

One of the most difficult aspects of pediatric nursing is coping with the death of a child. For nurses working in the pediatric intensive care unit (PICU), end-of-life care (EOLC) and pediatric deaths are often encountered. Each year, approximately 45,000 children (about twice the seating capacity of Madison Square Garden) ages 0 to 19 years die in the United States.[1] The largest decline in mortality rates since 1990 has been in children ages 5 to 9 years due to the decrease in the number of infectious diseases.[2]

[a] Louisiana State University Health Sciences Center-New Orleans, School of Nursing, 1900 Gravier Street, Room 5B14, New Orleans, LA 70112, USA; [b] Nicholls State University, School of Nursing, 906 East 1st Street, Thibodaux, LA 70301, USA
* Corresponding author.
E-mail address: bnwoko@lsuhsc.edu

Crit Care Nurs Clin N Am 35 (2023) 275–286
https://doi.org/10.1016/j.cnc.2023.04.002
0899-5885/23/© 2023 Elsevier Inc. All rights reserved.
ccnursing.theclinics.com

Although pediatric mortality rates are declining globally, many children experience death in the PICU after a planned withdrawal or limitation of life-sustaining treatment.[2] These events, coupled with a rigorous and complex environment, causes short- and long-term effects on health care workers such as decreased comfort level in providing EOLC, decreased job satisfaction, increased attrition rates, and burnout.[3,4]

Because of the negative impact of initiating EOLC to the pediatric population, organizations must be proactive in instituting education on EOLC and providing advanced skills to nurses who take care of patients at their EOL. The purpose of this article is to summarize the evidence on the impact of PICU nurses providing EOLC to their patients. This paper seeks to answer the question: what are the consequences of nurses providing EOLC in the PICU setting?

BACKGROUND
Pediatric Intensive Care Unit

The environment of the PICU setting is unique in that it provides experiences that cannot be found in many other areas of nursing. Patients of all ages are seen and cared for in the PICU, ranging from infants to teenagers, with varying diagnoses from incurable diseases to traumatic injuries.[5,6] Children are inundated with tubes, lines, and machines, battling pain, and frequently have several health care team members in the room and at their bedside. Compounding variables such as patient acuity, high-stake decisions, and intricate nursing skills can be overwhelming and inflict short- and long-term effects on both the patient's caregivers and health care providers.[7] The diverse characteristics of the PICU require nurses with specific expertise, which creates additional stressors.[3] The high-risk population of the PICU exposes nurses to EOLC and pediatric death, producing adverse effects such as uncertainty when performing skills or providing care, compassion fatigue, burnout, and decreased job satisfaction.[4] Moreover, the impact of the COVID-19 global pandemic on pediatric critical care nurses and its influence on their well-being has been well documented within the literature.[8] These working conditions have the potential to affect nurses working within the PICU specialty and, ultimately, the overall care received by the patients. Because of this, it is essential to evaluate what the literature states regarding these conditions and what can be done from an organizational and practice perspective to aid nurses at the bedside and offer high-quality, patient-centered care to this vulnerable population.

End-of-Life Care and Palliative Care

The terms EOLC and palliative care have been used interchangeably in the literature. Although the plans of care are different, the results of nurses performing EOLC or palliative care are similar. EOLC is defined as care of the patient as they near the EOL and includes physical, emotional, social, and spiritual care of the patient and their families.[9] Palliative care in its most simple explanation is care that focuses on enhancing the quality of life for patients and their families and offers additional holistic support as patients near the EOL.[10] Palliative care can last months or even years. Furthermore, palliative care focuses on accessing information and assisting with medical decision-making.[11] This article focuses on EOLC.

The death of a child may occur suddenly within minutes or days of the cause, whereas others occur days to years after an initial diagnosis or injury.[3,12] Regardless of the cause, comprehensive work is being done to understand the best practices in initiating EOLC in the PICU. According to the National Institutes of Aging,[13] EOLC should take a multidisciplinary approach inclusive of the whole patient, family, and care team with a focus on comfort, compassionate and clear communication, and psychosocial and spiritual support through the death life cycle. Unlike adults, children, particularly those unable to verbalize their needs (ie, age, cognitive level, and so forth) are unable to articulate their wishes when it comes to EOL decisions; this can be difficult for health care providers because they are often tasked with the need to inform and support the family.

Considering the number of tasks that a nurse performs during a shift with the addition of EOLC, the work environment can be physically and psychologically exhausting.[14,15] Carvajal and colleagues[16] reported that when nurses are charged with providing EOLC to patients, they are filled with heavy emotions such as stress, anxiety, overwhelmingness, and powerlessness. The weight of managing these emotions complicates an already taxing and understaffed nursing workforce. Although this environment seems difficult enough, the experience for nurses in a pediatric setting, caring for a child at the EOL can be exponentially worse.

Broden and colleagues[2] used a mixed method approach to examine the experiences of families with children who died in the PICU. Parents reported feelings of being overwhelmed, accounts of watching their children fight or struggle, and the competing difficulty of wanting to be with their children while allowing for the critical and complex care required. Similarly, Butler and colleagues[17] and Whyte-Nesfield and colleagues[18] examined the psychological stress that parents of EOLC patients are met with and described the parental traumatic stress that occurs because of a child's admission into the PICU. Using a combination of validated scales and questionnaires, Whyte-Nesfield and colleagues[18] assessed posttraumatic stress disorder (PTSD) and posttraumatic stress symptoms (PTSS) at 4 different time intervals (T0–T3), 3 to 14 days into admission, at discharge, 3 to 9 months postdischarge, and 18 to 30 months postdischarge. With a total of 265 patients meeting eligibility for the study, 14.8% and 12.5% met qualification for PTSD at 3 to 9 months and 18 to 30 months, respectively. In addition, 42% and 33.7% met criteria PTSS at 3 to 9 months and 18 to 30 months, respectively.[18]

Butler and colleagues[17] interviewed 18 bereaved parents. Throughout the interviews, the resonating themes included the importance of communication, the role of the parent and provider, and teamwork/collaboration between parents and health care provider. Gaining an understanding of parents' feelings of "handing over their child" and "nervousness about interfering with the provider's care" is an essential concern that influences the relationship between providers and parents and the way that providers administer the needed care of their patients. These parental feelings can greatly influence the health care provider's emotional well-being and patient outcomes.

Consequences of Pediatric Intensive Care Unit Nurses Engaging in End-of-Life Care

Several studies were examined to assess the consequences that providing EOLC had on nurses working with pediatric patients.[4,12,17,19,20] Throughout these studies, themes identified included communication challenges, nurse-family bonds, nursing resiliency, delivery of care challenges, discomfort with providing EOLC, and working through negative feelings.[4,6,12,20] In addition, Gagnon and Kunyk[19] cited moral distress and environmental constraints on nursing roles and responsibilities as being common themes associated with providing EOLC in PICUs.

Caring for patients at their EOL can be daunting and challenging for health care providers. Recognizing the barriers that nurses face when providing EOLC is important in creating healthy work environments and effective EOLC plans for patients who are dying. The following sections present the consequences of providing EOLC among nurses. These consequences include perceived comfort, nurse personal factors, compassion fatigue, burnout, moral distress, and lack of job satisfaction.

Perceived Comfort (Lack of Knowledge)

EOLC is an immense and traumatic experience for all involved. The daily nursing tasks, countless decisions, and interdisciplinary communication between health care providers and families ultimately affect everyone involved. These factors create an intense environment, often affecting communication among all parties. Nurses report feeling torn between decisions and carrying out plans of care, whereas caregivers are often left feeling torn between their roles.[5,17] Globally, there are more than 26 million men and women who make up the nursing workforce, accounting for approximately 50% of the total health care workforce.[21] With an overwhelming percentage of the workforce being nurses, equipping nurses with EOLC skills is critical. Because of this continuous and intimate involvement with patients, nurses must feel comfortable and confident in instituting EOLC. The comfort level of nurses providing EOLC is influenced by many factors such as EOLC education, therapeutic communication skills, workplace support, and prior history with providing EOLC.[5,22,23] Interestingly, there is a paucity of evidence on the comfort level of pediatric nurses providing EOLC.

Several studies found that despite ICU work experience, ICU nurses' attitudes toward caring for the dying patient were lower than most nurses working in other specialty areas.[22] On the other hand, Richoux and colleagues[24] found that nurses working in areas that frequently provided EOLC, such as the ICU and oncology units, have an increase in comfort and positive attitudes when providing care during the EOL than those working in other specialty units. Evidence also indicates a positive correlation between nurses receiving EOLC education and their comfort level in providing EOLC.[4,5,25] Exposure to EOL skills development and simulation on pediatric deaths enables nurses to discuss their feelings, debrief on their actions, and develop resiliency to overcome some of the challenges and negative impacts those situations may create.[5,12]

There has been much discussion about the preparation of nurses to provide EOLC. Although it seems that exposure to EOLC and pediatric deaths should, at least, be discussed within undergraduate or graduate curriculums, this is a component that is often missing from nursing programs' curriculums or only provided in small increments through various courses within the curriculum.[26–28] Several studies described new graduate nurse's preparation in prelicensure studies and found that new nurses are underprepared to provide EOLC to patients on graduation,[15,29–31] particularly among pediatric patients.[31,32]

Nurse Personal Factors

With the overwhelming emotional and psychological impact that nurses experience when caring for a patient at the EOL, there are many personal factors, such as social influences, spirituality, resiliency, and self-care, that influence a nurses' ability to provide EOLC. Personal factors are characteristics of an individual, such as gender, age, education, coping styles, social background, and experiences, which can affect functioning positively or negatively. These personal factors are not part of a health condition or health state.[33] Without an understanding of how to manage these personal factors, the ability for nurses to provide optimal care for themselves and patients can be negatively affected.

Personal factors are important to consider when considering how those caring for pediatric patients at the EOL perceive their experiences.[33] Social influences affecting the nurses' ability to provide EOLC relate to societal, organizational, and patient pressures that may be placed on nursing staff. These pressures create the expectation that nurses are trained to do this job and that they can manage this care and go on to the next patient with little or no recovery time. This can be a daunting expectation, especially for pediatric nurses.[20,34] Furthermore, for an impressive 20 years in a row, nursing has been the most trusted profession, according to a Gallup study.[35] Nursing as a trusted profession, may put nurses in a position to feel obligated to maintain this reputation in order to remain a strong and dependable profession in health care.

During this time of vulnerability in providing EOLC for patients and families, the nurse's role also involves providing spiritual care. Although it is an interdisciplinary approach with spiritual providers in the hospital, or of the family's choosing, nurses facilitate conversations and initiate resources to meet the patient and family's needs. This obligation may weigh on nurses religious and spiritual beliefs, causing increased distress and feelings of overwhelming emotions.[3,5,20]

As nurses navigate their personal factors influencing their ability to provide patient care, self-care is essential. In undergraduate nursing curriculums, there is much focus on nursing knowledge and skills, however, very little focus on the mental health and wellness of the nurse.[36] When nurses do not practice self-care or have effective coping mechanisms in place, they are vulnerable to negative repercussions such as burnout, decreased job satisfaction, and depression. The sadness and inability to disconnect their work trauma from their personal life when providing EOLC can gravely influence the mental health and wellness of nurses. Organizational support that includes training in resiliency and self-care can be helpful in promoting a healthy work environment.[4,20] Unfortunately, when health care organizations are not invested in the mental health and wellness of staff, staff are unable to balance their own personal factors and may be susceptible to negative outcomes, such as compassion fatigue.

Compassion Fatigue/Burnout

Compassion fatigue and burnout are considered contributing factors for nurses leaving the bedside and the profession altogether. It is estimated that 48% to 53% of nurses experience compassion fatigue.[37] Compassion fatigue is a phenomenon that has great impact among nurses regardless of their specialty area. It is correlated with individuals who work in highly challenging and complex environments that involve patients who are experiencing pain and suffering at their EOL.[38] These challenging and complex environments call for nurses to work at a faster pace, while making clinical decisions for multiple patients at the same time. Nurses tend to experience anxiety, depression, and even secondary traumatic distress because of the residue of caring for patients and their families when providing EOLC or after experiencing the death of a patient.[5,20] The vulnerability of the pediatric population compounded with the empathetic nature of the relationships formed between nurses and patients creates a nursing workforce susceptible to compassion fatigue and burnout.

Compassion fatigue is characterized as emotional exhaustion due to prolonged interaction with traumatized patients in high stressed environments. This emotional exhaustion can lead to numerous psychological and physical distresses.[37,38] Feelings of depression and anxiety have been tied to compassion fatigue within the pediatric nursing specialty.[20,39]

Although compassion fatigue and burnout are similar, they are not the same. According to the Nursing Advisory Board nurses report burnout as the number one reason for leaving their current employment. Burnout has been linked to the mismatch between the skills and preparation of workers and the job that they are expected to do. More importantly, burnout has been correlated with poor patient outcomes.

Burnout is defined as emotional exhaustion, depersonalization, and decreased productivity that typically occurs in the work environment.[38] A person experiencing burnout may feel hopeless, overwhelmed, inefficacy, unfulfilled with one's work, trapped, and have difficulty sleeping.[38,40] Burnout occurs 35% to 45% among United State nurses.[41]

Nevertheless, there are similarities between compassion fatigue and burnout. These similarities include emotional, physical, and mental exhaustion; isolation; and depersonalization.[38] Although compassion fatigue has a faster onset, burnout is much slower. It is important to note that compassion fatigue has a faster recovery when identified early.[38]

Because of empathetic patient engagement and inherent complexities of the relationships formed with families, pediatric nurses experience burnout differently from nurses working with adult patients.[8] These experiences affect the mental health and well-being of pediatric nurses.

Moral Distress

Moral distress is a situation that occurs when an individual knows the morally right thing to do but is hindered from taking the appropriate action because of internal or external limitations.[25,42] Critical care nurses are frequently exposed to seriously ill and at times terminally ill patients. Situations such as EOLC, medical futility, and periviable resuscitation can cause moral distress among health care providers.[25] The inability to alleviate patients' distress and the duty to deliver life-sustaining treatment can trigger moral distress. Similar to compassion fatigue, moral distress has contributed to burnout and job turnover or lack of job satisfaction.[42] **Fig. 1** illustrates a conceptual model of the consequences of EOL without proper resources and support.

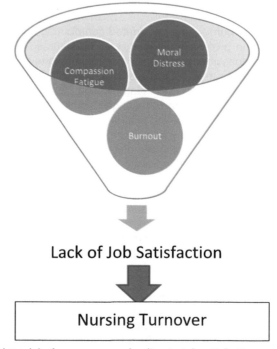

Fig. 1. Conceptual model of consequences leading to job satisfaction and nursing turnover.

Nursing Turnover

According to the American Association of Critical Care Nurses[43] health care professionals should preserve their personal morality and sense of justice to be effective in their work. Frequently, nurses are told to separate their emotions and just do their job. They adopt a stoic demeanor to maintain order, take care of their patients, and preserve the respect of their colleagues and loved ones. This act leaves damaging repercussions that can no longer be ignored in health care settings. Some signs and symptoms of moral distress include feelings of irritation, annoyance, and guilt. In addition, physical and psychological manifestations may happen. Some physical signs and symptoms include upset stomach, heart palpitations, lack of sleep, or weakness. Psychological signs and symptoms include withdrawal, emotional exhaustion, and depersonalization of patients.[43] **Figs. 2** and **3** depict what actions institutions should take to prevent moral distress and what support systems should be in place, respectively.

Furthermore, AACNb[43] recommends that nurses must act on their morals and recognize when it conflicts with what is being asked of them or what the situation may call for them to do. Other recommendations included seeking out a mentor; seeking and using a qualified mental health expert (ie, counselor, therapist, and so forth); and leaning on their colleagues, friends, and family.

Job Satisfaction/Nurse Turnover

There are a multitude of factors that contribute to the overall level of job satisfaction for nurses working at the bedside, regardless of specialty. Some of the most discussed components (**Fig. 4**) are contributed to economic, organizational, and personal factors.[44] Throughout this article, several of these aspects have been discussed, as they relate to nurses' ability to provide EOLC.

One of the most widely discussed economic factors across all workforces is pay. In a survey of more than 11,000 nurses, 68% stated that the most important thing their organization could do to increase overall work satisfaction would be to increase pay or offer bonuses (American Nurses Foundation, 2022). Although pay is not the most important aspect of a nurse's job, the compensation is an incentive for the expertise in skills and continual education that is expected of nurses, especially those in critical care settings. In addition, without adequate preparation and training, nurses feel ill-prepared to make decisions related to EOLC and are less confident in EOL skills.[19]

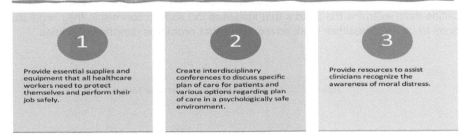

Fig. 2. Institutional actions against moral distress. (*Data from* American Association of Critical Care Nurses [AACNb]. AACN position statement: Moral distress in times of crisis. 2020. Available at: https://www.aacn.org/policy-and-advocacy/aacn-position-statement-moral-distress-in-times-of-crisis.)

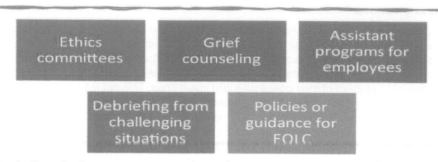

Fig. 3. Organization support systems. (*Data from* American Association of Critical Care Nurses [AACNb]. AACN position statement: Moral distress in times of crisis. 2020. Available at: https://www.aacn.org/policy-and-advocacy/aacn-position-statement-moral-distress-in-times-of-crisis.)

Adequate preparation and training are also associated with organizational support. Much of the training nurses receive postgraduation provided by the organization. These training courses are usually specific to the patient population and setting of the nurse.[45] In critical care, there is often a longer orientation, compared with acute care units with typical orientation lasting 12 to 14 weeks, and some organizations try up to 24 weeks in critical care orientation[46]; this is due to the increased levels of patient acuity and additional skills nurses need to optimally care for their patients, especially as it pertains to EOLC. Roberts and Doyle[47] reported the need for health care organizations to provide ongoing EOL education to assist nurses working in critical areas such as the PICU. The more that nurses feel supported within their work environment, the more confident they feel about obtaining clarity when practicing skills or making decisions.

As these environmental, organizational, and personal factors influence job satisfaction, research shows that job satisfaction directly affects nursing turnover (see **Fig. 1**).[48] The lack of appropriate training, such as EOLC can adversely affect job satisfaction among nurses caring for chronically ill children, leading to increased turnover.[49] The national nursing turnover rates have been continually increasing over the last few years. According to a report released by NSI Nursing solutions in 2022, using 2021 data collected from 272 hospitals, in 32 states, the national nursing turnover rate increased by 6.4% and is currently at an average of 25.9%, with ranges from 8.8% to 37.0% (NSI, 2022). Although this is the average rate, specific turnover rates vary by specialty and region. Increasing turnover rates often result in decreasing experience within these units, which leads to poor patient outcomes. Health care facilities must examine the factors that influence job satisfaction within their organizations to create a healthier work environment that promotes retention of nurses.

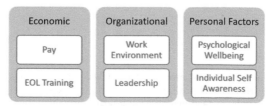

Fig. 4. Factors contributing to overall job satisfaction.

SUMMARY OF FINDINGS FOR FUTURE RESEARCH

The purpose of this article was to summarize the evidence on the impact of PICU nurses providing EOLC to their patients. According to our findings, several themes were identified as results of performing EOLC in the PICU. These included perceived comfort due to a lack of knowledge; influence of personal factors such as life experiences, age, education, and so forth; compassion fatigue; burnout; moral distress; and lack of job satisfaction. Because of the high incidences of exposures to death in the PICU, nurses working in the critical care environment should be well prepared to initiate EOLC. A lack of knowledge and skillset in performing EOLC can affect the mental health and wellness of nurses working in the PICU.[50] Each of these components leads to increasing attrition rates in an already diminished nursing workforce.

Key recommendations from the literature focused on the lack of EOLC education in schools of nursing and health care environments. The integration of EOLC curriculum into schools of nursing was highly regarded as a first step.[50] Nurses face dying and death among patients in various clinical settings, and schools of nursing will need to prepare a workforce that is prepared for these types of challenges. Several resources can be used by schools of nursing to provide additional content on EOLC. One example is the *End-of-Life Nursing Education Consortium* (ELNEC). ELNEC has EOLC information that can be used not only by clinicians but also by schools of nursing. In addition, the ELNEC project Web site has been updated to include more information to support the core competency *hospice/palliative/supportive care across the lifespan and with diverse populations*.[51] Roberts and Boyle[47] recommended that ongoing EOLC education within the clinical setting is important in meeting the needs of PICU nurses. These educational sessions should also include topics focused on mental health and wellness of nurses, palliative care and EOLC skillsets, and self-care strategies. Furthermore, there is a strong support in the literature for organizational support for nurses. This support from nursing and administrative leadership results in a feeling of appreciation and well-being, increasing the confidence and moral of nurses working within the organization. Effective organizational support includes work engagement strategies, open and receptive communication, and educational resources.[49] It also includes resources that focus on the mental health and well-being of nurses (see **Figs. 2** and **3**).

SUMMARY

Nurses play a significant role in caring for dying children. Many children spend their last days in the PICU setting. It is therefore important that PICU nurses attain the appropriate skills to create a supportive environment before, during, and after the time of death. However, evidence has shown that nurses do not have formal education or training in EOLC, leading to barriers such as moral distress, compassion fatigue, job dissatisfaction, and decrease in resiliency. Overcoming and understanding barriers of EOLC could greatly improve nurses' job satisfaction and attrition rates. It is necessary to institute formal EOLC curriculum or continuing education within schools of nursing and health care organizations.

CLINICS CARE POINTS

- The environment of the PICU setting is unique in that it provides experiences that cannot be found in many other areas of nursing.

- With the overwhelming emotional and psychological impact that nurses experience when caring for a patient at the EOL, there are many personal factors, such as social influences, spirituality, resiliency, and self-care, that influence a nurses' ability to provide EOLC.
- Environmental, organizational, and personal factors influence job satisfaction; research shows that job satisfaction directly affects nursing turnover.
- Ongoing EOLC education within the clinical setting is important in meeting the needs of PICU nurses.
- There is a strong support in the literature for organizational support to enhance mental health and wellness among nurses, particularly nurses working in critical patient care areas.

DISCLOSURE

The authors have nothing to disclose.

REFERENCES

1. Linebarger JS, Johnson V, Boss RD. Guidance for pediatric end-of-life care. Pediatrics 2022;149(5). https://doi.org/10.1542/peds.2022-057011.
2. Broden EG, Hinds PS, Werner-Lin A, et al. Nursing care at end of life in pediatric intensive care unit patients requiring mechanical ventilation. Am J Crit Care 2022; 31(3):230–9.
3. Mahon PR. A critical ethnographic look at paediatric intensive care nurses and the determinants of nurses' job satisfaction. Intensive Crit Care Nurs 2014; 30(1):45–53.
4. Küçükkelepçe GE, Özkan TK, Beşirik SA. The relationship between moral distress levels and ethical climate perceptions of PICU nurses. J Nurs Manag 2022;30(7):2416–23.
5. Poompan P, Fongkaew W, Mesukko J, et al. End-of-Life care for children and families in pediatric intensive care: Thai nurses' perspectives. Pacific Rim International Journal of Nursing Research 2020;24(3):335–48.
6. Broden EG, Deatrick J, Ulrich C, et al. Defining a "good death" in the pediatric intensive care unit. Am J Crit Care 2020;29(2):111–21.
7. Coats H, Bourget E, Starks H, et al. Nurses' reflections on benefits and challenges of implementing family-centered care in pediatric intensive care units. Am J Crit Care 2018;27(1):52–8.
8. Buckley L, Berta W, Cleverley K, et al. What is known about paediatric nurse burnout: a scoping review. Hum Resour Health 2020;18(1):9.
9. O'Shea ER, Lavallee M, Doyle EA, et al. Assessing palliative and end-of-life educational needs of pediatric health care professionals: results of a statewide survey. J Hospice Palliat Nurs 2017;19(5):468–73.
10. Pyke-Grimm KA, Fisher B, Haskamp A, et al. Providing palliative and hospice care to children, adolescents and young adults with cancer. Semin Oncol Nurs 2021;37(3):151166.
11. Rothschild CB, Derrington SF. Palliative care for pediatric intensive care patients and families. Curr Opin Pediatr 2020;32(3):428–35.
12. Mu PF, Tseng YM, Wang CC, et al. Nurses' experiences in end-of-life care in the PICU: a qualitative systematic review. Nurs Sci Q 2019;32(1):12–22.
13. Providing Care and Comfort at the End of Life. [NIH] National Institute on Aging NIA.

14. Ozga D, Woźniak K, Gurowiec PJ. Difficulties perceived by ICU nurses providing end-of-life care: a qualitative study. Glob Adv Health Med 2020;9. https://doi.org/10.1177/2164956120916176. 216495612091617.

15. Bloomer MJ, Ranse K, Butler A, et al. A national Position Statement on adult end-of-life care in critical care. Aust Crit Care 2022;35(4):480–7.

16. Carvajal A, Haraldsdottir E, Kroll T, et al. Barriers and facilitators perceived by registered nurses to providing person-centred care at the end of life. A scoping review. International Practice Development Journal 2019;9(2):1–22.

17. Butler AE, Copnell B, Hall H. The impact of the social and physical environments on parent–healthcare provider relationships when a child dies in PICU: findings from a grounded theory study. Intensive Crit Care Nurs 2019;50:28–35.

18. Whyte-Nesfield M, Kaplan D, Eldridge PS, et al. Pediatric critical care–associated parental traumatic stress: beyond the first year. Pediatr Crit Care Med 2023;24(2):93–101.

19. Gagnon M, Kunyk D. Beyond technology, drips, and machines: moral distress in PICU nurses caring for end-of-life patients. Nurs Inq 2022;29(2). https://doi.org/10.1111/nin.12437.

20. Kleis AE, Kellogg MB. Recalling stress and trauma in the workplace: a qualitative study of pediatric nurses. Pediatr Nurs 2020;46(1):5–10.

21. World Health Organization Nursing and midwifery. Nursing and Midwifery.

22. Fristedt S, Grynne A, Melin-Johansson C, et al. Registered nurses and under-graduate nursing students' attitudes to performing end-of-life care. Nurse Educ Today 2021;98:104772.

23. Kondo M, Nagata H. Nurses' involvement in patients' dying and death. Omega: J Death Dying 2015;70(3):278–300.

24. Richoux DN, Chatmon BN, Davis AH, et al. Factors impacting pediatric registered nurse attitudes toward caring for dying children and their families: a descriptive study. J Pediatr Nurs 2022;67:155–60.

25. Mills M, Cortezzo DE. Moral distress in the neonatal intensive care unit: what is it, why it happens, and how we can address it. Frontiers in Pediatrics 2020;8. https://doi.org/10.3389/fped.2020.00581.

26. Bahceli PZ, Donmez AA, Akca NK. Perceived barriers and motivators of under-graduate nursing students in end-of-life care: a qualitative study based on lived experiences. Psychiatr Care 2022;58(4):2687–96.

27. Rietze LL, Tschanz CL, Richardson HRL. Evaluating an initiative to promote entry-level competence in palliative and end-of-life care for registered nurses in Canada. J Hospice Palliat Nurs 2018;20(6):568–74.

28. de Campos AP, Walsh S. Nurses' degree of comfort in caring for palliative and hospice patients: a national survey. Medsurg Nurs 2021;30(6).

29. Baudoin CD, McCauley AJ, Davis AH. New graduate nurses in the intensive care setting. Crit Care Nurs Clin 2022;34(1):91–101.

30. Hao Y, Zhan L, Huang M, et al. Nurses' knowledge and attitudes towards palliative care and death: a learning intervention. BMC Palliat Care 2021;20(1):50.

31. Rawlings D, Winsall M, Yin H, et al. Holding back my own emotions": evaluation of an online education module in pediatric end-of-life care. J Child Health Care 2022. https://doi.org/10.1177/13674935221076214. 136749352210762.

32. Kadivar M, Mardani-Hamooleh M, Kouhnavard M, et al. Nurses' attitudes toward caring for terminally ill neonates and their families in Iran: a cross-sectional study. J Med Ethics Hist Med 2021. https://doi.org/10.18502/jmehm.v14i4.5651.

33. Grotkamp SL, Cibis WM, Nüchtern EAM, et al. Personal factors in the international classification of functioning, disability and health: prospective evidence. Aust J Rehabil Counsell 2012;18(1):1–24.

34. Stuart P. How do hospital nurses experience end-of-life care provision? A creative phenomenological approach. Br J Nurs 2022;31(19):997–1002.

35. Gaines K. Nursing Ranked as the Most Trusted Profession for 21st Year in a Row.; 2023.

36. Bernburg M, Groneberg D, Mache S. Professional training in mental health self-care for nurses starting work in hospital departments. Work 2020;67(3):583–90.

37. Chatmon BN, Rooney E. Taking care of the caretaker: navigating compassion fatigue through a pandemic. Aust J Adv Nurs 2021;38(3):1–4.

38. Kawar LN, Radovich P, Valdez RM, et al. Compassion fatigue and compassion satisfaction among multisite multisystem nurses. Nurs Adm Q 2019;43(4):358–69.

39. Arbios D, Srivastava J, Gray E, et al. Cumulative stress debriefings to combat compassion fatigue in a pediatric intensive care unit. Am J Crit Care 2022; 31(2):111–8.

40. Missouridou E, Mangoulia P, Pavlou V, et al. Wounded healers during the COVID-19 syndemic: compassion fatigue and compassion satisfaction among nursing care providers in Greece. Psychiatr Care 2022;58(4):1421–32.

41. National Academy of Medicine. In: Wakefield MK, Williams DR, Le Menestrel S, editors. The future of nursing 2020-2030: Charting a Path to achieve health equity. 2021.

42. Wolf AT, White KR, Epstein EG, et al. Palliative care and moral distress: an institutional survey of critical care nurses. Crit Care Nurse 2019;39(5):38–49.

43. American Association of Critical Care Nurses. AACN position statement: Moral distress in times of crisis.

44. Senek M, Robertson S, Ryan T, et al. Determinants of nurse job dissatisfaction - findings from a cross-sectional survey analysis in the UK. BMC Nurs 2020; 19(1):88.

45. Innes T, Calleja P. Transition support for new graduate and novice nurses in critical care settings: an integrative review of the literature. Nurse Educ Pract 2018; 30:62–72.

46. Miller J (2021, O 19). Rethinking Critical Care Orientation. Published online October 19, 2021.

47. Roberts KE, Boyle LA. End-of-Life education in the pediatric intensive care unit. Crit Care Nurse 2005;25(1):51–7.

48. Maunder RG, Heeney ND, Strudwick G, et al. Burnout in Hospital-Based Healthcare Workers during COVID-19.; 2021. doi:10.47326/ocsat.2021.02.46.1.0.

49. Diaz L. Leading through crisis: identifying ethical competencies for nurse leaders to effectively retain and support nurses in the era of COVID-19 within the United States. J Multidiscip Res 2023;15(1):137–41.

50. Subih M, Al-Amer R, Malak MZ, et al. Knowledge of critical care nurses about end-of-life care towards terminal illnesses: levels and correlating factors. INQUIRY: The Journal of Health Care Organization, Provision, and Financing 2022;59. https://doi.org/10.1177/00469580221080036. 004695802210800.

51. American Association of Colleges of Nursing [AACNa]. ELNEC expands resources for faculty on palliative and end-of-life care education.

Palliative Communication in the Pediatric Intensive Care Unit

Stevia Davis, MSN, PNP-PC, FNP[a],*,
Melissa Nunn, DNP, APRN, CPNP—PC/AC, CNE[b,c]

KEYWORDS

- Pediatric • Palliative care • Communication strategies • Discussions • Pediatric ICU
- Nursing

KEY POINTS

- Palliative communication with patients and families regarding their life-limiting illness is generally uncomfortable and most nurses believe ill-equipped to navigate these discussions.
- There are a variety of communication strategies that can be used to help mitigate the feeling of discomfort when discussing serious illness.
- The practical communication frameworks provided can be used to improve communication, establish and foster therapeutic alliances with the patients and their families.
- Communication is one of the most vital skills to possess and our communication skills need to be honed and practiced for the most effective and compassionate care.

INTRODUCTION
Pediatric Palliative Care Background

The World Health Organization defines palliative care (PC) as an approach to care that improves the quality of life of patients and their families facing the problems associated with life-threatening illnesses through the prevention and relief of suffering by means of early identification and assessment and treatment of pain and other problems: physical, psychosocial, and spiritual.[1] PC focuses on enhancing the quality of life and reducing suffering through relief of symptoms, integrating the psychological and spiritual aspects of care, and use of an interdisciplinary team. Pediatric PC (PPC) is known for its holistic approach in the care of patients and families facing

[a] Pediatric Palliative Care, Children's Hospital of New Orleans, 200 Henry Clay Avenue, ACC Suite 2020, New Orleans, LA 70118, USA; [b] Louisiana Health Science Center, New Orleans - School of Nursing; [c] Primary Care and Acute Care Concentrations
* Corresponding author.
E-mail address: stevia.davis@LCMChealth.org

Crit Care Nurs Clin N Am 35 (2023) 287–294
https://doi.org/10.1016/j.cnc.2023.04.003
0899-5885/23/© 2023 Elsevier Inc. All rights reserved.

serious illness.[2] PPC is family-centered and enhances quality of life, reduces suffering, and can help with communication and coordination of care.

It is important to discern the difference between PC, hospice care, and end-of-life care. PC can start at any time during a serious illness, whereas hospice care focuses on a person's final months of life. End-of-life care is the care that is delivered when the prognosis of death is almost certain and close in time.[2] PC can take place in conjunction with life prolonging or curative treatments; it does not depend on the course or stage of illness and can take place in intensive care unit (ICU) settings. Because PC can start from the time of diagnosis, pediatric ICU nurses often take care of PC patients throughout various stages in their illness trajectory, including when they are in the final months to moments of their illness lives. Although access to specialty PPC may be limited by geographic availability, hours of service, and limitations of team members, primary PPC is defined as training bedside clinicians the basic tenets of PPC.[2] Primary PPC training can help to reduce moral distress for nurses; a tenet of primary PPC training is effective communication.[3,4]

Nurses' Unique Role in Providing Primary Palliative Care

Nurses have the unique opportunity to play a pivotal role in their patient's care, especially when it comes to communication. Owing to the continuity of care nurses provide and the longevity of various disease processes that patients receiving PPC experience, nurses often develop longitudinal relationships with patients and families. As a nurse builds a relationship based on trust and consistency, they may be viewed as "more approachable" than others in the health care team.[5] With the relationship, nurses are generally the most trusted members of the care team and can provide unique insight into the patient, family, and their goals of care.

Barriers to Palliative Communication

Open and honest communication is an essential aspect of PPC. Communicating bad news is uncomfortable and is often avoided by nurses and other health care team members. However, delivering difficult information is a skill that can be learned and one that nurses innately possess due to the nature of the nursing role.

There are many barriers to providing open and honest communication regarding a child's life-limiting illness or impending death. A prominent barrier for health care providers is the stressful and uncomfortable nature of these conversations.[6] Often, in an effort to avoid discussing poor prognosis, clinicians will use optimist language and frequently wait for families to ask specific questions regarding prognosis; this hesitancy can lead to patients misjudging their chance of cure or life prolongation, which may impact their decision-making.[7]

Although most nurses do not feel adequately trained to participate in such discussions, nurses have the unique and pivotal opportunity to make a lasting impact on their patient/family's care plan as they are often key witnesses in the child's care.[8,9] By nature of their role, nurses bear witness to patients and families at their most vulnerable times, which can help foster the empathy essential for PC communication.

Goals of Palliative Communication

Most parents of children with life-threatening illnesses report a desire for disclosure of difficult information, such as poor prognosis or future limitations for their child.[2] Often, clinicians worry that disclosure of difficult information will be distressing and will deprive families of hope; however, studies have found that many parents consider prognosis communication to be both difficult and necessary.[10] Parents shared that while upsetting, prognostic information disclosure fostered hope by relieving uncertainty and allowing them to make the best possible decisions for their children.[11]

Communication is a central aspect of nursing care, especially in PC. All nurses can help to provide primary PC by using specific communication techniques that can help to elicit the patient and family's wishes when experiencing a life-limiting or life-threatening disease or event. The goal of these discussions is to help create a more complete depiction of the patient and family to understand their preferences and goals of care better. Ideally, goals of care discussions occur during periods of stability and calm. Because the nurse is at the bedside and likely has the most longitudinal interactions, they can engage in such discussions.

Advance care planning

Anticipatory guidance lays the foundation for exploring with the parent and, when possible, the child's preferences for their care as their condition changes. This information is then used to help inform advance care planning (ACP) over the course of the child's care. Anticipatory guidance is a necessary precursor to ACP.

When providing anticipatory guidance, it is essential to elicit and understand the patient/family's values which can be elicited by asking open-ended questions, referenced below. The benefits of ACP include preparation for end-of-life care, such as choosing death location preference, a decreased perception of suffering, and a better experience with end-of-life care.[12–14] Attending to patient and family preferences can promote rapport-building, trust, and shared decision-making over time. A goal of palliative communication is to understand the patient/family's goals of care and create a care plan that aligns with those goals.

Key questions to consider

1. What is your child like as a person? What is a good day like for your child?
2. What have you heard from the doctors about what is going on with your child?
3. How has this experience been for you and your child?
4. Given what you know about your child's disease, what is most important to you?
5. What are you hoping for? What else are you hoping for?
6. What worries do you have right now? What keeps you up at night?
7. Where do you find your strength? How well is that support working for you right now?
8. What else should I know about your child/your family to take the best care of you?

These communication techniques can be especially helpful when transitioning care plans from cure to comfort and quality of remaining life. It can be uncomfortable to transition from discussions focused on cure to discussions focused on quality of life and comfort, the communication tools provided below can aid in dissipating some of the discomfort and stress of these conversations.

CLINICS CARE POINTS

- NURSE: repsonse to patient and family emotions
- SPIKES: delivering difficult communication
- Ask-tell-ask: open communication

COMMUNICATION TOOLBOX

NURSE (responding to patient and family emotions)[5,15]:

Naming the emotion assures the patient of the nurse's recognition of the patient/family's emotion
- "You seem really upset since the doctor talked with you this morning"
- "I can see how overwhelmed you are."

Understanding using words that communicate understanding normalizes the patient's emotion with a nonjudgmental attitude.
- "It is understandable to feel overwhelmed."
  *Avoid suggesting that you understand what they are feeling, instead try "I can't imagine how you are feeling, but it wouldn't surprise me if you were feeling sad right now" this helps the patient/family to know the nurse understands that they are having a difficult time

Respect: Communicating respect acknowledges the patient's ability to overcome some of the challenges of his/her life-limiting illness. It shows acknowledgment of the challenges that the patient is encountering and coping with:
- "Anyone in your shoes would feel overwhelmed right now."
- "You are doing a great job despite how overwhelming it is."

Support: Using words that communicate support communicates the nurse's presence at that time and in the future, assuring the patient/family of non-abandonment. Making this kind of commitment is a powerful statement
- "I will support you as best I can"
- "I know you have been struggling with pain. I will continue to work with you to control this problem and help you reach your goals."
- "I will do my best to find answers to your questions, so that the next steps feel less overwhelming."

Explore: The nurse can communicate empathy through words that explore his/her experience.

Exploring creates space for the patient and family to talk about what they are going through and can help to explore the values behind decisions and potential sources of conflict.
- "Tell me more. What overwhelms you the most right now?"
- "When you say you feel [xxx], what do you mean?"

Ask-Tell-Ask[5,16]: This allows for open and appropriate communication based on the family's wishes. This tool allows you to assess how much the patient and family know, how much they want to know, and how much they wish to discuss it. When using this approach, questions should be open-ended to determine the needs and allow further discussion. For example, "What have you heard about...", "Here is what the tests show...", "Does this make sense to you?" and "What questions do you have?"
    SPIKES (delivering difficult news)[5,17]:

Setting up and Starting: Mentally rehearse and arrange for privacy
- Find a quiet location
- Invite important family and friends to be present
- Have tissues readily available
- Turn off your phone/ringer off
- Have enough chairs for everyone
- Introduce everyone in the room
- Acknowledge and reflect on your own discomfort

Perception: Elicit the patient/family's perspective
- Determine what the patient and family already knows
  - "What have you heard about your child's condition?"
  - "What have your doctors told you about your child's illness?"
  - "What is your body telling you?"
  - "How have you seen your child's body changing?"
- Look for and affirm knowledge and emotional information during response
  - "You have a very good understanding of the situation."
  - "I can sense how frustrating this experience has been for you."
- *Do not interrupt

Invitation: Ask the patient what they would like to know about the diagnosis, prognosis, and details about their illness or treatment options.
- Explore how much information the patient and family want to know
  - "Some families like to hear all of the details. Others prefer to get the big picture summarized for them. How do you like to hear medical information?"
- Ask for permission to discuss difficult topics
  - "Is it okay if we talk about some changes I am seeing?"
  - "Would it be okay if I discuss X with you?"

Knowledge: Provide information in small pieces
- Use a "warning statement" to help the patient and family emotionally prepare
  - "I'm really sorry to say that we have bad news today."
  - "I have something serious we need to discuss."
- Give the information simply and clearly. Avoid medical jargon. Give small bits of information and then stop.
  - "I have noticed her breathing has changed and I worry she is actively dying."
- Ask-Tell-Ask

Emotions: Recognize and empathize with patients/family's emotions
- Respond to emotion: affirm, normalize, support
  - "This must be shocking to hear."
  - "I can't imagine how difficult this is."
  - "I can see that you are angry. This is awful and unfair, and you have every right to feel this way."
  - "Every parent (or patient) feels frightened when they hear bad news like this. You are not alone. We will help guide you every step of the way."
  - "It is normal to feel upset and overwhelmed. It's ok to take things 1 hour at a time."
- Silence is golden: wait quietly for the patient and/or family to process and emote in their own way and time

Strategy and *Summary*: Set out a medical plan of action
- Discuss next steps and follow-up plan
  - "We just talked about a lot of information. I know this can feel overwhelming. Is it ok if I summarize what we just talked about?"
  - "Let's go over the plan for the coming week again, to make sure that you know what to expect."
- Secure a lifeline
  - "If you have worries or questions or need to talk to someone, you can call this number (or send a message through this portal, etc.)"

When you get stuck

Silence

Tell me more…

I wish, I worry, I wonder

I Wish, I Worry, I Wonder

I wish allows us to align with a patient or family's hopes while also addressing the limits of treatments[18]. *I worry* allows us to be truthful while being sensitive. It shares concern without stating certainty that something will or will not occur. *I wish* and *I worry* statements can often be used together and help to recognize that families are often holding hopes while also holding worries. For example, when a child is nearing end of life, we may use "I also wish that [parent hope] were possible, and I also worry that time is short." *I wonder* helps to demonstrate empathy and allows us to make a gentle recommendation.

I Wish Statements
- "I wish that things were different, it isn't fair"
- "I wish we had a chemotherapy treatment that would cure your child's cancer"
- "I wish that I had better news to tell you."

I Worry Statements
- "I worry that the chemotherapy treatment will not work"
- "It's very hard to talk about what may happen if treatment doesn't work. If we don't discuss this, I worry that you and your family won't be prepared if things don't go the way we hope."

I Wonder Statements
- "I wonder if now is an okay time to talk about next steps?"
- "I wonder what is most important to you/your child. What things would you want to focus on? How would you like to spend most of your time? Where would you want to be?"
- "I wonder if there are some options that we haven't considered that we could explore?"

Terms/Phrases to Avoid

Although learning helpful phrases and terminology to use in PC is important, it is also essential to be aware of terms and phrases to avoid. We often use shortcuts in our language when discussing patients and prognosis with other team members, and we often bring that language into our conversations with families. This can result in misunderstanding between what we say and what is heard, resulting in two different understandings.

What is said versus patient/family perception	
What Health Care Provider Says	**What Patient/Family Hears**
His creatinine is better.	He will get well.
She is stable today.	She will get better.
We have an experimental treatment	This new therapy will cure my child
Do you want us to use CPR?	You think CPR will help
Do you want us to "do everything" for your child?	Doing everything means you think my child will survive and get well.

Curative versus palliative: This terminology is often used with disease directed treatment and suggests that only two outcomes are possible, when in reality, the outcomes are more nuanced.[2] Families often hold multiple "intents" or "hopes" for disease directed therapy.[19] *Transitioning to palliative care/redirecting care/do nothing* these terms all imply that something new is being offered. PC is not a phase of care but rather an integrated approach to care throughout a serious illness trajectory. *Doing nothing* should never be suggested as we are always doing something for the patient, and we never stop caring for the patient or family. *Withdrawal or withholding of support/care* is often inferred by parents as stopping all care rather than discontinuing a particular intervention; for example, "discontinuation of life sustaining therapies with an intensive focus on supportive care." When described as withdrawal or withholding, parents may think that their child will no longer receive care and is often isolating. *The child failed:* for example, *"the child failed extubation"* implies that the child was at fault for the intervention not succeeding, when truly no one has failed.

Helpful phrases for communication	
Unclear/Distressful Language	**Helpful Language**
It's time to pull back	Let's think about/discuss discontinuing treatments that are not providing benefit or causing more symptoms
There is nothing more we can do	We may consider changing the goals of care Let's review the goals of care to see if any of them have changed
A miracle may turn things around	In my experience, I have not seen a child in this situation survive.

SUMMARY

Communication is a complex process that should be individualized. Nurses have a unique role in advocating for the child and family's best interests. Through tailored communication techniques, nurses have the opportunity to guide families in choosing care plans that are in line with their goals of care. The various communication strategies presented can be added to the nurse's communication toolbox to aid them in navigating these critical scenarios. Communication is a learned and vital skill that requires listening, openness, flexibility, and practice to aid in delivering effective and compassionate care.

DISCLOSURE

The author has no conflict of interest.

REFERENCES

1. WHO Definition of Palliative Care. Available at: https://www.who.int/news-room/fact-sheets/detail/palliative-care. Accessed February 5, 2022.
2. Wolfe J, Hinds P, Sourkes BM. Interdisciplinary pediatric palliative care. 2nd edition. Oxford University Press; 2022.
3. Lafond DA, Bowling S, Fortkiewicz JM, et al. Integrating the comfort theory into pediatric primary palliative care to improve access to care. J Hosp Palliat Nurs 2019;21(5):382–9.
4. National Academies of Sciences, Engineering and Medicine, Health and Medicine Division, Board on Health Sciences Policy, Board on Health Care Services. Rountable on quality care for people with serious illness. *Models and Strategies to integrate palliative care Principles into Care for People with serious illness: Proceedings of a workshop.* Washington, DC: The National Acadamies Press (US); 2017.
5. Peereboom K, Coyle N. Facilitating goals-of-care discussions for patients with life-limiting disease – communication strategies for nurses. J Hosp Palliat Nurs 2012;14(4):251–8.

6. Studer RK, Danuser B, Gomez P. Physicians' psychophysiological stress reaction in medical communication of bad news: a critical literature review. Int J Psychophysiol 2017;120:14–22.
7. Mack JW, Fasciano KM, Block SD. Communication about prognosis with adolescent and young adult patients with cancer: information needs, prognostic awareness, and outcomes of disclosure. J Clin Onc 2018;36(18):1861–7.
8. Lafond DA, Kell KP. End-of-life decision making in pediatric oncology. In: Ferrell BR, Paice JA, editors. Oxford textbook of palliative nursing. 5th edition. New York: Oxford Press; 2005. p. 736–48.
9. McDaniel C, Desai JM. Pediatric goals of care: leading through uncertainty. In: Ferrell BR, Paice JA, editors. Oxford textbook of palliative nursing. 5th edition. New York, NY: Oxford Press; 2019. p. 727–35.
10. Nyborn JA, Olcese M, Nickerson T, et al. "Don't try to cover the sky with your hands": parents' experiences with prognosis communication about their children with advanced cancer. J Pall Med 2016;19(6):626–31.
11. Boss RD, Lemmon ME, Arnold RM, et al. Communicating prognosis with parents of critically ill infants: direct observation of clinician behaviors. J Perinatol 2017;37(11):1224–9.
12. Curtis Jr, Patrick DL, Engelberg RA, et al. A measure of the quality of dying and death. J Pain Symptom Manage 2002;21(1):17–31.
13. Mack JW, Weeks JC, Wright AA, et al. End-of-life discussions, goal attainment, and distress at end of life: predictors and outcomes of receipt of care sonsistent with preferenes. J Clin Oncol 2010;28(7):1203–8.
14. Decourcey DD, Silverman M, Oladunjoye A, et al. Advance care planning and parent-reported end-of-life outcomes in children, adolescents, and young adults with complex chronic conditions. Crit Care Med 2019;47(1):101–8.
15. Fischer G, Tulsky JA, Arnold R. Communicating a poor prognosis. In: Portenoy R, Bruera E, editors. Topics in palliative care. New York: Oxford Press; 2000.
16. Back AL, Arnold RM, Baile WF, et al. Approaching difficult communication tasks in oncology. CA Cancer J Clin 2005;25(6):57–64.
17. Baile WF, Buckman R, Lenzi R, et al. SPIKES—a six-step protocol for delivering bad news: application to the patient with cancer. Oncol 2000;5(4):301–11.
18. Partain DK, Strand JJ. Common challenges in a palliative medicine consultation. In: Robinson MT, editor. Case studies in neuropalliative care. Cambridge (United Kingdom): Cambridge University Press. p. 8–12.
19. Bluebond-Langer M, Belasco JB, Goldman A, et al. Understanding parents' approaches to care and treatment of children with cancer when standard therapy has failed. J Clin Oncol 2007;25(17):2414–9.

Unplanned Extubation in the Pediatric Intensive Care Unit

Julianne Moss, MS, CPNP-AC[a,b,*], Brieann Maurer, MSN, CPNP-AC[a],
Cynthia Howes, MS, CPNP-AC[a]

KEYWORDS

- Unplanned extubation • Pediatric intensive care unit • Endotracheal intubation
- Mechanical ventilation • Critically ill children • Reintubation • Quality improvement

KEY POINTS

- Unplanned extubation (UE) in the pediatric intensive care unit is a common complication of endotracheal intubation.
- The rate of UE is a patient safety and quality of care measure.
- UE can increase morbidity and mortality in critically ill children.
- Staff identification of patients at risk for UE and when UE occurs is important for patient outcomes.
- Implementation and adherence of an UE bundle are effective in decreasing the rate of UE.

INTRODUCTION

Unplanned extubations (UEs) in the pediatric intensive care unit (PICU) are a common, potentially avoidable complication of endotracheal intubation among infants, children, and adolescents. The rate of UEs in the PICU is both a patient safety and quality of care measure. Recent pediatric studies have reported the incidence of UE in the PICU to be 0.4 to 0.77 events/100 intubation days.[1-9] Earlier studies have reported a wider range and higher incidence of UE (0.4–6.4 events/100 intubation days) among PICUs and a higher incidence (4.0 events/100 intubation days) among the neonatal ICU (NICU) population.[5,10,11] As high as 65% of patients who experienced an UE require reintubation, leading to increased days of mechanical ventilation (MV), longer PICU stay, and increased risk of life-threatening complications.[4] Quality improvement (QI) initiatives including the implementation of UE bundles, staff education, and standardization of care have been shown to decrease the incidence of UE.[1,7,10]

[a] Department of Pediatric Critical Care, University of Maryland Children's Hospital, 22 South Greene Street, Baltimore, MD 21201, USA; [b] University of Maryland Children's Hospital, 110 South Paca Street, 8th Floor, Baltimore, MD 21201, USA
* Corresponding author. University of Maryland Children's Hospital, 110 South Paca Street, 8th Floor, Baltimore, MD 21201.
E-mail address: Julianne.Moss@som.umaryland.edu

Crit Care Nurs Clin N Am 35 (2023) 295–301
https://doi.org/10.1016/j.cnc.2023.04.004
0899-5885/23/© 2023 Elsevier Inc. All rights reserved.

Care of the mechanically ventilated infant and child poses a unique challenge to intensive care providers due to inherent differences of the pediatric airway and their developmental immaturity. It is important to note that tracheal diameter and length increase with age making the need for proper positioning of an endotracheal tube (ETT) in a pediatric airway more precise.[12] Small manipulations in endotracheal depth can result in extubation or right mainstem bronchus intubation, both of which can result in patient decompensation. Prompt recognition of a malpositioned ETT relies on careful and constant assessment by the bedside staff in order to prevent patient harm.

Additionally, inconsistent practices in sedation and muscle relaxation in pediatric patients receiving MV could affect the rate of UE. A wide range of variability among sedation regimens for children requiring MV has been reported.[13] The American College of Critical Care Medicine (ACCM) recently published comprehensive clinical practice guidelines that address sedation, analgesia, and delirium management of critically ill children.[13] Administration of intermittent narcotics, benzodiazepines, and use of paralytics an hour before UE event was found to be statistically significant in a study conducted by Al-Albdawni and colleagues.[1] Additionally, Censoplano and colleagues found that inadequate sedation and agitation was a contributing factor in half of the UEs.[5] This evidence may suggest inadequacies in the baseline level of sedation before UE events and highlights an area where QI efforts in the PICU can be focused. Bedside staff is responsible for assessing the level of sedation and notifying providers when adjustments in medications are required. A patient safety incident such as an UE is a reviewable event that should lead to changes in practice, preferably through a multi-disciplinary QI project.

CURRENT EVIDENCE

UEs in the PICU lead to increased hospital length of stay, MV days, need for reintubation, and an overall increase in hospitalization costs.[3–5,7,8,14] Roddy and colleagues found that an UE was associated with a longer PICU length of stay (10 vs 4.5 days), longer hospital length of stay (16.5 vs 10 days), and a higher total cost of hospitalization (US\$101,310 vs US\$64,618).[8] This demonstrates a significant financial impact similar to that reported for catheter-associated bloodstream infections (US\$33,000 to US\$55,000 per sentinel event).[8] Additionally, UE events can cause significant respiratory and cardiovascular instability in pediatric patients, including hypoxemia, bradycardia, and cardiac arrest. Al-Abdwani and colleagues reported that up to 53% of UE cases experienced adverse events, including cardiac arrest (2%), bradycardia (11%), and stridor (14%).[1] Da Silva and colleagues found a higher mortality rate for patients who experienced an UE.[3] The significant impact of UEs on morbidity and mortality for hospitalized children in the PICU demonstrates the immense need for recognizing high-risk patients, environmental and staffing factors, critical review of UE events and tailored QI initiatives to reduce their incidence.

Complications following an UE often depend on the severity of the underlying illness but multiple studies have identified risk factors for UE independent of diagnosis. The most common risk factors identified for UE are agitation or inadequate sedation, poorly secured ETT, and younger than 1 year of age. See **Table 1** for a full list of risk factors.[1,3,5,9,15,16,18,19] Not only is it essential for PICU staff to be able to identify patients who are at risk for UE but it is also equally important to recognize patients who will likely need reintubation following an UE for clinical preparedness. Risk factors for reintubation include patients aged younger than 1 year, need for full MV support, longer duration of MV, increased oxygen requirement, higher oxygenation index, lower Pao_2/Fio_2 ratio, copious secretion amount, as well as a deeper level of sedation and/or

Table 1	
Risk factors for unplanned extubation	
Patient Factors	**Staff/Environmental Factors**
• Agitation/Level of sedation[3,5]	• Nurse–patient ratio >1:2[3]
• Continuous sedation infusion[3]	• Nurse/RT experience <2 y[1,3]
• Oxygenation index > 5[3]	• Night shift[3]
• Inadequate ETT securement[5]	• Weekend shift[1]
• Age <1 y[5,15,16]	• Frequent hand off of care[1]
• Lack of physical restraint[1]	• Repositioning/transport[15,16]
• Oral intubation[5,15]	• Patient procedures[15]
• Copious secretions[17]	• Prone positioning[16]
• Difficult airway[9]	
• Uncuffed ETT[5,18]	

recent administration of benzodiazepine or muscle relaxant.[1,3,4,20] As many as one-third of patients who require reintubation have significant cardiovascular and respiratory complications.[4] In a long-term study by Censoplano and colleagues, 20% of patients who were reintubated required cardiopulmonary resuscitation, with one patient needing mechanical circulatory support.[5] Identifying patients at risk for reintubation following an UE can prepare staff to respond promptly and appropriately to decrease morbidity.

Alternatively, not every patient who experiences an UE requires reintubation. Da Silva and colleagues found that 73% of patients who were in the process of weaning MV toward extubation and experienced an UE did not require reintubation.[2] Similar findings in other studies suggest that medical teams often fail to identify when a patient is clinically ready for extubation.[1,8] There is a need for further research in pediatrics to determine the optimal timing for extubation.

RECOGNITION OF UNPLANNED EXTUBATION

Knowing the most vulnerable patients and the highest risk times for UEs is important for bedside staff; however, they must also be able to identify when an ETT has been displaced. An UE can be observed directly or radiographically as dislodgement of the ETT from the airway. Nursing education can significantly improve quick recognition, and assessment of equal breath sounds on auscultation, presence of expiratory waveforms on the ventilator, appropriate capnography during manual ventilation, and color change on an end-tidal CO_2 detector decreasing amount of time until UE is recognized.[17] Checking the integrity of the ETT securement with each patient assessment is important in identifying when an ETT needs to be resecured. Sudden changes in vital signs such as hypoxia, bradycardia, or tachycardia and loss of end-tidal CO_2 in a patient with an ETT should alert the medical staff of a possible UE. If a patient has an UE, bedside staff should provide advanced airway management through bag-mask ventilation until other PICU staff arrives to assist.

Once an UE has occurred, the PICU team must then assess the patient and determine if reintubation is needed or if noninvasive respiratory support measures can be used to support the patient. Noninvasive options can be considered in patients as a bridge to possibly delay the need for reintubation in the form of high-flow nasal cannula or noninvasive positive pressure ventilation (NIPPV) encompassing bilevel positive airway pressure, or continuous positive airway pressure. According to Abdel-Rahim and colleagues, up to 83.3% of patients successfully used NIPPV to wean from MV without the need for reintubation in a PICU.[21] Patients with decreased level of consciousness, higher oxygen index, or difficulty with secretion management should be recognized quickly because of an increased risk for reintubation, and staff should prepare necessary medications and equipment.[3]

REDUCTION OF UNPLANNED EXTUBATION

In recent years, QI initiatives have been successful in decreasing the rate of UEs in a variety of studies.[17,18,21–24] Many of these initiatives have focused on staff education, environmental restructuring, guidelines, and communication.[15,18,23] In a meta-analysis of 11 studies, implementation, and adherence to a UE bundle has shown to reduce the incidence of UE by 60%.[2] Klugman and colleagues showed a 17% to 24.1% reduction in UE events with their bundle in a multi-center study.[7] There has also been improvement in UE events in low-resourced PICUs with the utilization of a low-cost bundle, which could have a potentially global impact in reducing pediatric morbidity and mortality.[18] Bedside staff participation in reviewing critical events can bring to attention the factors leading to the event, such as patient agitation or inadequate sedation, poorly secured ETT, and staffing concerns.

When developing a bundle, it should be applicable to all intensive care units regardless of patient population and be sustainable over time. Based on the current evidence, bundle components should include standardization of ETT care, identification of high-risk patients, targeted sedation assessments, sedation standardization/protocolization, and readiness for extubation guidelines.[3,13] Vats and colleagues developed a risk assessment tool that successfully identified patients at high risk for UE, decreasing the rate of UE events in their PICU.[9] Utilizing a tool to identify patients at high risk of UE can allow the PICU to implement practice changes to decrease UE. Standardization of ETT care includes the use of cuffed ETT tubes, suctioning protocols, and securement/resecurement practices.[17,18] Currently, there is no gold standard for ETT securement; nevertheless, when a unit standardizes their practice for ETT securement, it can lead to a decrease in UE. Nasotracheal intubation should be considered when clinically appropriate because it has been shown to have a lower rate of UE in pediatric cardiac patients aged younger than 2 years.[22] Working with nurses and respiratory therapists, a PICU should create standardized ETT practices based on their patient population and identified issues in the review of critical events.

The ACCM recommends the use of protocolized sedation and that all pediatric patients requiring MV have assigned a target depth of sedation using a validated sedation assessment tool at least once daily.[13] Routine use of the COMFORT-B Scale or the Richmond Agitation-Sedation Scale to assess the level of sedation in mechanically ventilated patients may help identify patients who are not appropriately sedated.[13] Additionally, identification of delirium through assessment tools such as the preschool and pediatric confusion assessment methods for ICU or the Cornell Assessment for Pediatric Delirium and appropriate treatment could reduce UEs.[13] Targeting a depth of sedation, sedation weaning protocol, standardized securement, and adjusting nursing workload to facilitate more frequent monitoring have been recommended to decrease UE in the time surrounding a planned extubation.[13] Each unit should review its critical events to tailor their UE bundle. It is critical that staffs are invested and adhere to the bundle to decrease the rate of UE, or else the bundle will not produce the desired effect. See **Fig. 1** for a sample QI bundle.

CONTROVERSIES

Varying definitions of UE and inconsistent interpretation of UE events may contribute to underreporting and the wide range in reported incidence. Terms such as "self-

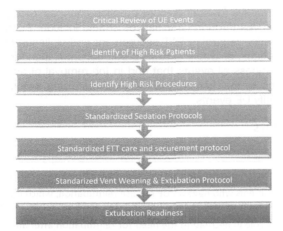

Fig. 1. Components of QI bundle.

extubation," when an ETT is dislodged by a patient either deliberately or unintentionally with patient activity implies patient responsibility and should be avoided because it does not capture all UE events such as those caused by staff manipulation or urgent removal by staff in response to patient decompensation. Al-Abdwani and colleagues propose a more all-encompassing definition of UE, which comprises all events in which "displacement or removal of an ETT occurs at a time other than that specially chosen for a planned extubation."[1] Other inconsistencies in reporting of UE include events that occur in the ICU versus those that occur outside of the ICU whether on transport or in the operating room and events in which the ETT is completely dislodged or externalized versus dislodged in the esophagus. In a study conducted by Ndakor and colleagues, using a less inclusive definition of UE, including only those described as "self-extubation" and occurring in the NICU resulted in 83% of events being excluded.[11] Due to the significant adverse effects associated with UE events, it is recommended that a comprehensive definition be utilized to categorize all nonelective extubations to better capture events that can be critically reviewed.

Risk factors for UEs varied among the studies; agitation, lack of sedation, improper ETT securement, and age less than 1 year were the most consistent. Although the evidence in regard to nursing staff ratios has been supported, and there are limited data in regard to time of day and transport. Some research suggested that the level of experience of bedside nursing was a factor in UEs; nevertheless, there are limited supporting data.[3,25] Each PICU will have individualized risk factors unique to their unit staffing, infrastructure, patient population, and so forth that increase the potential for UEs. This could suggest why conflicting data exist concerning UE risk factors in the current literature. A multidisciplinary review of UE events is essential for determining unit-specific risk factors and guiding practice changes.

SUMMARY

UE in the PICU is the most frequent patient safety event in children with artificial airways that can be prevented. Pediatric patients who have an UE are likely to experience respiratory and cardiovascular complications and require longer MV days and length of stay in the PICU, while ultimately increasing the financial burden of the health-care system. Identification of PICU patients at risk for an UE and at risk for reintubation is imperative for staff to start practice changes to decrease the rate of UEs. Prevention of UEs through QI initiatives should include a critical review of UE events, staff education regarding ETT securement and vigilance of at-risk patients, particularly during times of weaning toward extubation. A standard definition of UE is needed to encompass all events that end in the removal of an ETT that was not planned in advance by the medical team. By standardizing definitions, units will be able to better identify UE events.

CLINICS CARE POINTS

- UE is the most common preventable airway patient safety event in PICUs.
- Over half of the patients who have an UE require reintubation, which increases their risk of morbidity and mortality as well as their hospital stay and hospitalization costs.
- NIPPV may have a role in decreasing the need for reintubation after an UE.
- Implementation of UE bundles through QI initiatives can decrease the rate of UE in PICUs
- Core components of an UE include identification of high-risk patients, standardization of ETT care, and protocolized sedation.

DISCLOSURE

The authors of this article declare no conflicts of interest.

REFERENCES

1. Al-Abdwani R, Williams CB, Dunn C, et al. Incidence, outcomes and outcome prediction of unplanned extubation in critically ill children: an 11year experience. J Crit Care 2018;44:368–75.
2. da Silva, P., Reis, M. E., Farah, D., et al (2022). Care bundles to reduce unplanned extubation in critically ill children: A systematic review, critical appraisal and meta-analysis. Archives of Disease in Childhood, 107(3), 271– 276. Available at: https://doi-org.proxy1.library.jhu.edu/10.1136/archdischild-2021-321996.
3. da Silva, P., & Fonseca, M. (2020). Factors associated with unplanned extubation in children: A case-control study. Journal of Intensive Care Medicine, 35(1), 74– 81. Available at: https://doi-org.proxy1.library.jhu.edu/10.1177/0885066617731274.
4. da Silva P, Reis ME, Fonseca TSM, et al. Predicting reintubation after unplanned extubations in children: art or science? J Intensive Care Med 2018;33(8):467–74.
5. Censoplano N, Barrett C, Ing R, et al. Achieving sustainability in reducing unplanned extubations in a pediatric cardiac ICU. Pediatr Crit Care Med 2020; 21(4):350–6.
6. Kanthimathinathan HK, Durward A, Nyman A, et al. Unplanned extubation in a paediatric intensive care unit: prospective cohort study. Intensive Care Med 2015;41(7):1299–306.
7. Klugman D, Melton K, Maynord PO. Assessment of an unplanned extubation bundle to reduce unplanned extubations in critically ill neonates, infants, and children. JAMA Pediatr 2020;174(6):e200268.
8. Roddy DJ, Spaeder MC, Pastor W, et al. Unplanned extubations in children. Pediatr Crit Care Med 2015;16(6):572–5.

9. Vats A, Hopkins C, Hatfield KM, et al. An airway risk assessment score for unplanned extubation in intensive care pediatric patients. Pediatr Crit Care Med 2017;18(7):661–6.

10. Razavi SS, Nejad RA, Mohajerani SA, et al. Risk factors of unplanned extubation in pediatric intensive care unit. Tanaffos 2013;12(3):11–6.

11. Ndakor S, Pezzano C, Spilman L, et al. Wide variation in unplanned extubation rates related to differences in operational definitions. J Patient Saf 2022;18(1):e92–6.

12. Nichols DG, Rogers MC. Rogers' textbook of pediatric intensive care. 4th edition. Philadelphia: Lippincott Williams & Wilkins; 2008.

13. Smith HAB, Besunder JB, Betters KA, et al. 2022 society of critical care medicine clinical practice guidelines on prevention and management of pain, agitation, neuromuscular blockade, and delirium in critically ill pediatric patients with consideration of the ICU environment and early mobility. Wolters Kluwer Health 2022. https://doi.org/10.1097/PCC.0000000000002873.

14. Agarwal S, Classen D, Larsen G, et al. Prevalence of adverse events in pediatric intensive care units in the United States. Pediatr Crit Care Med 2010;11(5):568–78.

15. Wollny K, Cui S, McNeil D. Quality improvement interventions to prevent unplanned extubations in pediatric critical care: a systematic review. Syst Rev 2022;11:259.

16. Zhang P, Liu LP. Validation of a risk assessment tool for unplanned endotracheal extubation: an observational study. Clin Nurs Res 2022;31(8):1438–44.

17. Hatch LD, Rivard M, Bolton J, et al. Implementing strategies to identify and mitigate adverse safety events: a case study with unplanned extubations. Jt Comm J Qual Patient Saf 2019;45(4):295–303.

18. Jayawardena ADL, Ghersin ZJ, Guzman LJ, et al. A low-cost educational intervention to reduce unplanned extubation in low-resourced pediatric intensive care units. Int J Pediatr Otorhinolaryngol 2021;149(1). https://doi.org/10.1016/j.ijporl.2021.110857.

19. Fitzgerald RK, Davis A, Hanson SJ. MS3 national association of children's Hospitals and related institution PICU Focus Group investigators. Multicenter analysis of the factors associated with unplanned extubation in the PICU. Pediatr Crit Care Med 2015;16(7):e217–23.

20. Chang TC, Cheng AC, Hsing SC, et al. Risk factors for reintubation and mortality among patients who had unplanned extubation. Nurs Crit Care 2022;1–7. https://doi.org/10.1111/nicc.12777.

21. Abdel-Rahim M, Attia T, Abdel-Rahman D. Non-Invasive Ventilation in Preventing Intubation and Reintubation in The Intensive Care Unit of Pediatrics Zagazig University Hospital. Egypt J Crit Care Med 2020;81(7):2422–8.

22. Christian C, Thompson N, Wakeham M. Use and outcomes of nasotracheal intubation among patients requiring mechanical ventilation across U.S. picus. Pediatr Crit Care Med 2020;21(7):620–4.

23. Kaufman J, Rannie M, Kahn MG, et al. An interdisciplinary initiative to reduce unplanned extubations in pediatric critical care units. Pediatrics June 2012;129(6):e1594–600.

24. Meregalli CN, Jorro Barón FA, D'Alessandro MA, et al. Impact of a quality improvement intervention on the incidence of unplanned extubations in a Pediatric Intensive Care Unit. Arch Argent Pediatr 2013 Oct;111(5):391–7 [English, Spanish].

25. Marcin JP, Rutan E, Rapetti PM, et al. Nurse staffing and unplanned extubation in the pediatric intensive care unit. Pediatr Crit Care Med 2005;6(3):254–7.

Hematologic and Oncologic Emergencies in the Pediatric Intensive Care Unit

What Nurses Should Know.

Danielle Sebbens, DNP, CPNP-AC/PC[a,b,]*,
Jessica L. Spruit, DNP, CPNP-AC, CPHON, BMTCN[c]

KEYWORDS

- Hem/onc nursing • PICU nursing • Pediatric brain tumors • Pediatric stroke
- Pediatric oncologic emergency • Pediatric acute chest syndrome

KEY POINTS

- Nurses have a critical role in recognizing and continuously assessing children experiencing a hematologic or oncologic emergency.
- An understanding of the pathophysiology of a hematology/oncology diagnosis helps nurses focus their assessments and promptly respond to emergent symptoms.
- Nurses with training and experience caring for children admitted with hematologic or oncologic emergencies improve patient outcomes.[1]

INTRODUCTION

Caring for children in the pediatric intensive care unit (PICU) with a hematology/oncology (hem/onc) diagnosis is complicated and challenging. Nurses with training and experience caring for children admitted with a hem/onc emergency improve patient outcomes.[1] Neurological assessment skills, including Glasgow Coma Scale (GCS), motor strength, and pupil response, are essential for detecting decompensation in patients with brain tumors and stroke. Frequent evaluation of airway, breathing, and circulation, including heart rate, perfusion, and blood pressure, is vital for patients with a mediastinal mass, superior vena cava syndrome, acute chest syndrome (ACS), and febrile neutropenia (FN). Close monitoring for cardiac arrhythmia associated with

[a] Arizona State University, Edson College of Nursing and Health Innovation, 500 North 3rd Street, Phoenix, AZ 85004-0698, USA; [b] Phoenix Children's Hospital, 1919 East Thomas Road, Phoenix, AZ 85016, USA; [c] Mott Children's Hospital, 1540 East Hospital Drive, Ann Arbor, MI 48109, USA
* Corresponding author. Arizona State University, Edson College of Nursing and Health Innovation, 500 North 3rd Street, Phoenix, AZ 85004-0698.
E-mail address: dsebbens@asu.edu

Crit Care Nurs Clin N Am 35 (2023) 303–314
https://doi.org/10.1016/j.cnc.2023.04.005
0899-5885/23/© 2023 Elsevier Inc. All rights reserved.
ccnursing.theclinics.com

electrolyte derangement and strict measurement of intake and output is needed for children at high risk for developing tumor lysis syndrome (TLS). Early recognition and intervention for a decompensating pediatric hem/onc patient improve morbidity and mortality.[2] This article will review the pathophysiology/epidemiology, therapeutic options, and nursing considerations for patients admitted to the PICU with hem/onc emergencies associated with a brain tumor, stroke, FN, TLS, mediastinal mass/superior vena cava syndrome, and ACS.

Brain Tumor

Pathophysiology/epidemiology Brain tumors are the most common solid tumors in childhood. The incidence varies based on patient age, sex, race, ethnicity, and geography.[3] In the United States, between 2012 and 2016, the average annual adjusted incidence rate of all pediatric brain and other central nervous system (CNS) tumors (malignant and nonmalignant) was 6.06 per 100,000 children aged younger than 20 years.[3] Of these, 58% of the tumors were malignant.[4] Symptoms at the time of presentation depend on the patient's age and the tumor's location (**Table 1**).[5–7] Children of all ages may present with nonspecific, vague, or intermittent symptoms. Headache is the most common overall complaint.[5] Infants may have a bulging fontanel, macrocephaly, irritability, sunsetting phenomenon, and vomiting.[6,7] Older children may have more focal symptoms such as headache, nausea, vomiting, cranial nerve deficits, including visual deficits and anisocoria, and motor deficits, such as ataxic gait.[5–7]

Emergent presentations are primarily seen in patients with increased intracranial pressure (ICP). This increase in pressure can be caused by the tumor or hydrocephalus from the obstruction of the normal outflow of cerebrospinal fluid (CSF).[6,7] Oncologic emergencies associated with brain tumors can occur with initial presentation or related to acute treatment, for example, surgical intervention.[8] Symptoms associated with an increased ICP include headache, macrocephaly or bulging fontanel, nausea, vomiting, visual deficits, ataxia, irritability or behavior changes, and seizure. Early recognition of these symptoms, implementation of nursing interventions to decrease ICP, and notification of the appropriate providers may reduce the risk of long-term disability.

Therapeutic Options

Managing a pediatric brain tumor requires an interprofessional team of specialists for the best outcome. When the child presents with increased ICP, this team may include providers from pediatric critical care, neurosurgery, oncology, neurology, radiology, child life, palliative care, and social work.[5]

After the initial computed tomography (CT) scan of the brain is complete and increased ICP is confirmed, either from mass effect or from obstructive hydrocephalus,

Table 1	
Presentation of brain tumor and location[5–7]	
Presentation	**Location**
Seizures, weakness, muscle twitches/tremors, trouble speaking	Cerebral cortex
Anorexia, weight loss, growth failure	Hypothalamic
Visual/cranial nerve deficits	Occipital
Ataxia, fine motor dysfunction, balance disorders, vomiting, hydrocephalus	Cerebellar/posterior fossa
Balance disorders, cranial nerve deficits	Brainstem

the pediatric neurosurgeon may choose tumor resection, tumor biopsy, or placement of an external ventricular drain, if needed, to drain the CSF obstruction.[7] The goal of surgery is to remove the tumor entirely or perform a biopsy if resection is not possible while minimizing complications of bleeding, herniation, stroke, and morbidity or neurological deficits from injury to adjacent anatomy.[5]

MRI is ideal for evaluating, diagnosing, and long-term surveillance of brain tumors. Emergency presentation of a brain tumor with an increased ICP will delay MRI until after surgery. A contrast MRI should be obtained within 72 hours of the surgery to evaluate the surgery and CSF drainage and confirm the remaining tumor's absence.[7]

Additional treatment following surgical resection depends on brain tumor classification, which is difficult with pediatric brain tumors because they often contain multiple cell types.[6] Pediatric oncologists prescribe therapy based on tumor characteristics and national or international protocols. These therapies may include chemotherapy, radiation, targeted therapies, immunotherapy, antiangiogenic therapies, and other novel procedures.[7]

Nursing Considerations

Immediate nursing interventions for a patient with symptoms of increased ICP include elevating the head of the bed (HOB) to 30°, aligning the head and the neck in a neutral position, decreasing environmental stimulation, and limiting vagal maneuvers, including suctioning. Activate the rapid response team and call the responsible provider for the patient. Continue close monitoring for the development of Cushing triad, which includes bradycardia, hypertension, and irregular breathing.

Anticipate an immediate CT scan of the head. If the patient is unstable, the provider will prescribe therapies to stabilize the patient for transport. These may include hyperosmolar therapy with mannitol or hypertonic saline infusion. Moreover, anticipate giving intravenous dexamethasone, providing oxygen, maintaining normothermia, normoglycemia, normal or elevated blood pressure to enhance cerebral perfusion pressure, and frequent neurological assessments. Airway protection may be indicated for GCS less than 8 or if the patient has irregular breathing.

Pediatric Stroke

Pathophysiology/epidemiology. Pediatric stroke can be divided into categories based on age or by underlying cause, ischemic or hemorrhagic. A perinatal stroke occurs from 28 weeks gestation to 28 days postnatal, and a childhood stroke occurs after 28 days to 18 years of age.[9] This article will not include epidemiology or management of perinatal stroke. Ischemic stroke can be further defined by arterial ischemic stroke (AIS), venous infarction from cerebral sinovenous thrombosis, or cortical vein thrombosis.[9] The incidence of ischemic stroke in Western developed countries is 1 to 2 in 100,000 children.[10] Variability is seen with age and sex, with the highest incidence in children aged younger than 5 years, boys, and Black and Asian children.[11] The increased risk in black children is associated with sickle cell disease (SCD). Hemorrhagic strokes account for one-half of pediatric strokes, with an incidence of 1 to 1.7 in 100,000 per year.[9]

The most common symptoms of stroke in children mimic those in adults and are hemiparesis and hemifacial weakness (67%–90%), speech/language disturbance (20%–50%), visual disturbance (10%–15%), and ataxia (8%–10%).[9,12,13] Children may also have nonlocalizing symptoms such as headache (20%–50%) and altered mental status (17%–38%).[9] Children are more likely to present with a diagnosis that can mimic strokes, such as seizures, migraines with aura, or syncope.[9,13] AIS from cardiac disease occurs in children (median age 6 months to 3 years) more often in the inpatient setting.[9] Despite similar symptoms to adults, there are significant delays in detecting pediatric stroke, with one estimate up to 24 hours after the onset of symptoms.[9,13] Accurate and timely diagnosis by providers impacts morbidity and mortality, and diagnosis within 4.5 hours of symptom development is ideal for children to have the best outcome.[12]

Therapeutic options. In the United States, interprofessional teams and specialized facilities have been established as primary stroke centers for adults, resulting in rapid IV thrombolytic therapy (tPA) and endovascular thrombectomy.[12] The landmark Thrombolysis in Pediatric Stroke study was organized to establish protocols to allow tPA treatment of children.[14] Stroke teams were formed, and algorithmic pediatric stroke screenings led to an organized approach to treatment.[12]

The interprofessional stroke team is activated when a child presents with symptoms that could represent a stroke. MRI is more sensitive than a CT scan for the detection of pediatric stroke.[13] A head CT could identify an acute hemorrhage but could be normal in AIS. An MRI with diffusion-weighted imaging (DWI), magnetic resonance angiography (MRA) of the head and neck, and magnetic resonance venography (MRV), specifically if there is a concern for cerebral venous sinus thrombosis (CVST), to evaluate the stroke further.[13,15] Antithrombotic therapy can be initiated once a hemorrhagic stroke has been excluded. Following patient stabilization, further family history, laboratory testing, and possibly imaging will attempt to determine the underlying cause of the stroke and prevention of reoccurrence.

Nursing considerations. All health-care team members should remain vigilant and have an increased awareness of the manifestations of pediatric stroke. Although the incidence is relatively rare, the associated morbidity and mortality can be devastating. Early identification and activation of the stroke team improve outcomes. Perform age-based neurological assessments and share concerns with the interprofessional team. Anticipate the need for MRI with DWI, MRA, and MRV if the child's screening is positive. Qualification for tPA does not change the need for neuroprotective measures for stroke management. The mnemonic STROKE can help nurses remember the primary therapies for neuroprotection (**Box 1**).[16] Keep the HOB flat for 24 to 72 hours to improve cerebral perfusion pressure unless the increased ICP is a symptom.[13] Maintain euvolemia with fluid at a maintenance rate or at 1.5 times maintenance, avoid hyponatremia, prevent fever by using acetaminophen or a cooling blanket, avoid hypoglycemia and significant hypertension, minimize vasospasm by maintaining magnesium greater than 2, and monitor for/prevent seizures.[13]

Febrile Neutropenia

Pathophysiology/epidemiology. FN is an oncologic emergency.[17–20] Neutropenia is the term to describe an absolute neutrophil count (ANC) of less than 500 neutrophils/mm.[3]

Box 1
Stroke mnemonic[16]

S–Seizures

T–Temperature (Avoid fever)

R–Rest (Head of bed flat)

O–Over hydrate

K–Keep open and flowing (Systolic BP and anticoagulation)

E–Electrolytes (Glucose 100–160, Sodium >140, Magnesium>2)

Courtesy of A. Bucci, DNP, CPNP-AC, Phoenix Children's Hospital, Inc.

ANC is calculated by multiplying the total white blood cell count (WBC) by the (% neutrophils + bands). In patients with neutropenia, it is generally accepted that a fever is defined as a single episode of a temperature greater than 38.3° or a temperature for more than 1 hour of greater than 38°. In the United States, from 2007 to 2014, there were 104,315 admissions for FN.[18] There were more hospitalizations in 5 to 14-year-old boys of all races in the Midwest and Western hospital regions.[18] Overall mortality remained low, with the 15 to 19-year-old age group at greater mortality risk.[18] Patients with FN and sepsis, pneumonia, meningitis, or mycosis had the most significant mortality risk.[18]

Therapeutic options. The evaluation of a patient with FN begins with a detailed history and physical examination. The history should include details about the underlying oncologic diagnosis, last chemotherapy, and current medications.[19] Fever is not always caused by an infection in an oncology patient. They may have a reaction, allergy, or hypersensitivity to a recent medication. Medications may have a known side effect of fever. Blood product transfusion or graft versus host disease can also cause fever. Initial laboratory evaluation often includes a complete blood count (CBC) with differential, a comprehensive metabolic panel, and blood cultures. The need to obtain peripheral blood cultures remains controversial. Yet, a strong recommendation is to obtain cultures from all lumens of a central venous catheter based on international pediatric-specific guidelines.[19] Depending on the history, urine and stool cultures may be recommended. A chest radiograph is not universally recommended unless the patient has symptoms of an upper respiratory pathologic condition.[19] Empiric antibiotic therapy varies by patient's history of resistant organisms, presentation, and institutional antibiograms.[21] Anaerobic, antifungal, or antiviral therapy may also be considered. If there is a concern for sepsis, with or without shock, follow sepsis guidelines for patient care and appropriate resuscitation measures. Although there is interest in improving risk stratification and potentially treating patients at low risk as outpatients, the trend has continued to include hospitalization of all oncology patients with fever and neutropenia.[10]

Nursing considerations. A known treatment goal for treating patients with FN and the presence of a central venous catheter is to administer antibiotics within 60 minutes of their arrival at the hospital.[21] Nursing recognition of these high-risk patients can help reduce the time from arrival to admitting, obtaining laboratory tests, blood cultures, and administering antibiotics.[21]

Tumor Lysis Syndrome

Pathophysiology/epidemiology. TLS is one of the most common oncologic emergencies. TLS occurs when cancer cells break down and intracellular components are released into the bloodstream. Tumor cells may begin breaking down spontaneously before the cancer diagnosis or on the initiation of cytotoxic therapy, including chemotherapy or radiation. The metabolic derangements that result from the lysis of tumor cells place the pediatric patient at greater risk for severe complications, including acute kidney injury, cardiac arrhythmias, seizures, and death.[22,23]

This emergency is more common in hematologic malignancies such as leukemia and non-Hodgkin lymphoma due to the rapid cellular turnover in these tumors compared with solid or CNS tumors.[22] It is difficult to estimate the incidence of TLS in children with cancer due to the historical lack of unifying diagnostic criteria.[23,24] There are several factors to consider when determining the risk of a child developing TLS. Patients with malignancies with high-proliferation rates, such as acute lymphoblastic leukemia and Burkitt lymphoma, and those with high tumor burden in the form of bulky tumors or a significantly elevated WBC, are at increased risk.[23,24]

Tumors that are very sensitive to chemotherapy, radiation, or steroids are also at higher risk of TLS.[22,23] Underlying renal insufficiency and dehydration increase the risk of developing TLS-related complications.[8,23]

Therapeutic options. The diagnosis of TLS is made based on laboratory values or clinical presentation (Table 2).[22,25,26] A metabolic panel will be obtained to evaluate for hyperuricemia, hyperphosphatemia, hyperkalemia, and hypocalcemia. The presence of 2 or more of these metabolic derangements fulfills the criteria for laboratory TLS.[25,26] Although not part of the diagnostic criteria, the LDH will likely be elevated and is an important consideration when considering the patient's risk of TLS.[23] Clinical TLS is diagnosed when a patient has an elevated serum creatinine of 1.5× or greater the upper limit for age, cardiac arrhythmia or sudden death, and seizure.[22,25,26] Laboratory TLS is observed more often than clinical TLS.[27]

An interprofessional approach, including the oncology, nephrology, and critical care teams, is often required. Children at risk for TLS must be identified and monitored closely to prevent and minimize the complications of this oncologic emergency. Aggressive IV hydration will be initiated carefully to avoid complications associated with fluid overload.[22,23] Loop diuretics may be prescribed to optimize urine output.[22] Laboratory values will be obtained as frequently as every 4 hours depending on the risk and trends in results, especially as therapy is initiated.[23]

Treatment will address each of the electrolyte abnormalities present. Hyperuricemia may be prevented with allopurinol and treated with rasburicase.[23,24] There are several strategies to decrease serum potassium in hyperkalemia. Potassium is shifted into cells when insulin or beta-adrenergic agnostics such as albuterol are administered.[23] Loop diuretics and sodium polystyrene sulfonate promote excretion in the urine and stool, respectively.[23] In the setting of cardiac dysrhythmias secondary to hyperkalemia, calcium gluconate should be administered immediately to stabilize the cardiac membrane.[23,24] Hyperphosphatemia is prevented with dietary restrictions and hyperhydration. If preventive strategies are ineffective, phosphate binders, diuretics, and dialysis may be indicated.[23] Calcium is not administered except in the case of dysrhythmias due to the risk of calcium precipitation in tissues and kidney injury.[24] The risk of TLS typically resolves approximately 3 days after the initiation of chemotherapy.[23]

Nursing considerations. Nurses caring for children at risk for developing or currently being treated for TLS will closely monitor fluid status with frequent, accurate measurement of intake and output, weights, and monitoring for symptoms of fluid overload or dehydration.[22] Due to the risk of cardiac dysrhythmias during ongoing cellular breakdown and risk for hyperkalemia, continuous cardiac monitoring should be applied and

Table 2 Tumor lysis syndrome[22,25,26]	
Laboratory findings	Elevated • Phosphorus • Potassium • Uric Acid Decreased • Calcium
Clinical manifestations	Cardiac • Cardiac arrhythmia Kidney • Serum creatinine (>1.5× upper limit for age) Neurologic • Seizures

monitored for peak T waves and/or QRS widening.[23] Frequent blood draws will be required. If a child receives rasburicase for hyperuricemia, subsequent laboratory specimens are immediately placed in an ice bath to be transported to the laboratory due to the risk of inaccurate results secondary to ex vivo enzymatic lysis of uric acid in the laboratory vial.[23,28]

The nurse caring for a child with TLS is not only responding to a child and family during an emergency but in the setting of a new cancer diagnosis. Providing education regarding the need for strict and accurate intake and output, low potassium and phosphorus diets, and expectations during this critical time will help families process the significant amount of information they are receiving.

Anterior Mediastinal Mass

Pathophysiology/epidemiology. Anterior mediastinal masses are an oncologic emergency due to the cardiopulmonary consequences associated with compression of the airways and vasculature.[8,29] In the presence of an intrathoracic mass, the trachea and bronchi may be compressed or obstructed and predispose the patient to respiratory failure.[29] Decreased pulmonary perfusion and right-sided heart failure may result from pulmonary artery compression.[29] Pulmonary edema and decreased cardiac output are consequences of pulmonary vein compression.[29] Compression of the vasculature, heart, and great vessels increases the risk of cardiovascular collapse.[29] When the superior vena cava is compressed, there is an increase in venous pressure and decreased venous return increasing the risk for thrombosis, cerebral edema, and hemodynamic instability.[29,30] Clinical manifestations of an anterior mediastinal mass impacting the airway include cough, difficulty breathing, wheezing, stridor, hoarse voice, and difficulty swallowing.[8] Facial swelling may result from impaired venous return in the superior vena cava.[8,30] Retention of carbon dioxide may result from an anterior mediastinal mass, leading to changes in mental status (confusion, lethargy, anxiety), headache, visual disturbances, and syncope.[8]

Approximately 70% to 75% of mediastinal masses in children are malignant.[31] Certain pediatric oncologic diagnoses are associated with anterior mediastinal masses, including non-Hodgkin lymphoma, Hodgkin lymphoma, T-cell lymphoblastic leukemia, and less often, germ cell tumors, thymomas, and thyroid tumors.[8,29,32] Approximately 50% to 70% of children diagnosed with lymphoblastic lymphomas have a mediastinal mass at the time of diagnosis.[32] Among patients with anterior mediastinal masses, there is an estimated 5% to 20% risk of life-threatening complications secondary to anesthesia.[29,32]

Therapeutic options. Patients with an anterior mediastinal mass have a guarded airway and must be approached with extreme caution to preserve their respiratory and cardiovascular function. Interprofessional collaboration between specialists in critical care, oncology, anesthesia, interventional radiology, pediatric surgery, otolaryngology, and radiation oncology can promote the safe assessment and management of children with anterior mediastinal masses.[29] Diagnosis of a mass and the impact on surrounding tissues may be made by using two-view chest radiographs, chest CT, and echocardiogram.[8,29] A note of the patient's difficult airway may be placed within the electronic medical record and indicated in the patient's room for awareness in the event of an emergency. A biopsy of the tumor will guide disease-directed therapy but poses additional risks related to anesthesia.[32] General anesthesia could lead to decompensation secondary to loss of muscle tone, the collapse of airways, and further compression of cardiovascular structures.[32] Hemodynamic compromise may be worsened by reduced ventricular preload related to positive pressure ventilation during anesthesia.[32] To avoid general anesthesia, diagnosis of malignancy may be made by flow cytometry of peripheral blood or pleural fluid.[31] Mediastinal masses due to leukemia may be diagnosed with the evaluation of blasts in the peripheral blood.[31] Additional laboratory evaluations, including a CBC, review of morphology, metabolic panel, coagulation studies, and inflammatory markers may also aid in diagnosing and treating complications.[29] Treatment of the malignancy may include chemotherapy, radiation therapy, immunotherapy, targeted therapy, and other novel interventions per the guidance of pediatric oncologists.

Nursing considerations. Patients with a high-risk mediastinal mass often require critical care.[33] Caring for a child with a mediastinal mass should include very close observation of cardiorespiratory status with the goal of maintaining spontaneous respirations. Nurses should be prepared for emergent intubation, mechanical ventilation, and extracorporeal life support for children at high risk for collapse.[33] Children should be allowed to maintain a position of comfort as diagnostic evaluation is coordinated and performed. The collaboration of several specialists will promote the best outcomes and reduce the risks associated with medical interventions. Urgent administration of steroids or administration of radiation therapy may be required.[8]

Acute Chest Syndrome

Pathophysiology/epidemiology. SCD is the most common inherited blood disorder and there are an estimated 70,000 to 100,000 Americans living with the disease.[34,35] SCD is present at birth and is the result of abnormal polymerization of the hemoglobin molecule, leading to altered red blood cell (RBC) shape, increased adhesion molecules, and rapid hemolysis.[35,36] Sickling and hemolysis of RBCs lead to an inflammatory cascade in the endothelium and endovasculature causing acute and chronic organ damage.[36] Sickling of RBCs is promoted by dehydration, inflammation, infection, fever, and hemostasis.[37] SCD is more prevalent in people of African descent, Hispanic Americans from Central and South America, and people of Middle Eastern, Asian, Indian, and Mediterranean descent.[34]

There are several acute complications of SCD, including vaso-occlusive pain crisis, ACS, infection, stroke, acute anemia, splenic sequestration, and priapism.[35,37] ACS was originally described in 1979 to describe pneumonia-like events involving chest pain, cough, fever, an abnormal respiratory examination, and a new infiltrate on a chest radiograph in patients with SCD.[38] ACS is the second most common cause of hospitalization in patients with SCD.[38] It is estimated that approximately one-half of the patients with SCD will develop ACS, which accounts for approximately 25% of SCD deaths.[38] Patients with comorbid conditions of asthma and obstructive sleep apnea are at an increased risk of ACS.[38,39]

Therapeutic options. In the United States, newborn screening identifies infants at risk for SCD.[36] A laboratory test called hemoglobin electrophoresis, which quantifies the amount of hemoglobin S present in the blood, is performed to confirm the diagnosis.[35,36] Health maintenance strategies are essential in preventing and early recognition of complications related to SCD.[36] Asplenia increases the risk for invasive infection, requiring education, penicillin prophylaxis, and pneumococcal vaccination to reduce associated morbidity and mortality.[36] Screening with transcranial Doppler evaluations is used to identify patients at greater risk for stroke.[36] Triggers for vaso-occlusive crises should be identified and avoided, and pathways to address pain should be developed for patients with SCD. Patients with SCD may require pharmacologic therapy such as hydroxyurea or chronic exchange transfusion therapy per the guidance of their hematologist. Children with severe complications of SCD may be eligible for hematopoietic stem cell transplantation. Ongoing efforts to develop gene therapy or genetic reengineering may lead to a permanent cure in the future.[36]

A new infiltrate on chest imaging in addition to at least 2 clinical symptoms, including pleuritic chest pain, hypoxemia, tachypnea, or fever is defined as ACS.[35] Patients with ACS often present with fever, cough, shortness of breath, chest pain, and increased work of breathing.[37,38] ACS may be triggered by an infection or a painful vaso-occlusive pain crisis.[37,38] Although patients may present to the emergency department with these symptoms, ACS may also develop within one to 3 days of hospitalization for a vaso-occlusive pain crisis or in the postoperative period.[38] Empiric antibiotics and beta-agonist inhalation treatments are often prescribed due to the risk of ACS secondary to infection and bronchospasm, respectively. Supportive care, including adequate analgesia and incentive spirometry, will promote comfort and recovery from ACS by decreasing splinting and increasing tidal volume.[36,37] Supplemental oxygen therapy and transfusion, whether simple or exchange, can promote oxygen-carrying capacity.[37] Some patients with ACS will require critical care for advanced respiratory support, including a high-flow nasal cannula, noninvasive positive-pressure ventilation, and mechanical ventilation.[37]

Nursing considerations. Maintaining a high index of suspicion and awareness of the risks of ACS is critical for timely recognition and treatment. The interprofessional team caring for children with SCD and ACS may include the hematologist, pulmonologist, and critical care specialists. Assessment of work of breathing can alert the interprofessional team to the development or progression of ACS. Identification and intervention for pain with the encouragement of incentive spirometry every 2 hours is recommended.[37] Addressing pain is essential as the patient is encouraged to take deep breaths and participate in other recommended activities to prevent the progression to ACS during hospitalization. Nurses caring for children with ACS can engage child life or other supportive care services to promote age-appropriate deep breathing exercises and the use of spirometry. Arterial blood gases with co-oximetry are considered the gold standard for measuring blood oxygen content and may be more accurate, especially in patients with concerns of severe anemia or vaso-occlusive events where the accuracy of pulse oximetry has been questioned.[38] Hydration status will be closely monitored with the goal of euvolemia.[37] Simple transfusion with RBCs or exchange transfusion where some blood is removed, and then a transfusion is administered to decrease the percentage of hemoglobin S RBCs will be performed depending on the hemoglobin.[37,38]

SUMMARY

PICU nurses have an important role in the recognition and response to children experiencing a hematologic or oncologic emergency. Astute observation skills and excellent communication will enhance outcomes for these patients. The stress of instability, a new diagnosis, possible malignancy, and anticipation of surgery can have lasting psychological impacts.[7] The nurse has an invaluable role in supporting patients and families during an emergency and as they process information regarding a new diagnosis that will affect the lives of their entire family. Nurses are best positioned to recognize distress experienced by the child and family and advocate for interventions to support them, including engaging child life therapists, spiritual care, social work, psychology, and palliative care services as appropriate.

CLINICS CARE POINTS

- The astute observation skills of PICU nurses are required to recognize children experiencing a hematologic or oncologic emergency.

- Nurses with training and experience caring for children admitted with hematologic or oncologic emergencies improve patient outcomes.[1]
- Immediate bedside nursing interventions, for example, adjusting the head of bed, providing prescribed antibiotics within 60 minutes of arrival, close cardiorespiratory monitoring, strict intake and output, and administration of prescribed pain medications improve outcomes.

DISCLOSURE

The authors have nothing to disclose.

REFERENCES

1. Moussa AAH, Maaz AUR, Faqih N, et al. Critically ill pediatric oncology patients: what the intensivist needs to know? Pediatric Critical Care Medicine. Indian J Crit Care Med 2020;24(12):1256–63.
2. Cawood S, Bassingthwaighte M, Naidu G, et al. Outcomes of pediatric oncology patients admitted to an intensive care unit in a resource-limited setting. J Pediatr Hematol Oncol 2022;44(3):89–97.
3. Ostrom Q, Cioffi G, Gittleman H, et al. CBTRUS statistical report: primary brain and other central nervous system tumors diagnosed in the United States in 2012–2016. Neuro Oncol 2019;21(5):v1–100.
4. Fahmideh MA, Scheurer ME. Pediatric brain tumors: Descriptive epidemiology, risk factors, and future directions. Cancer Epidemiol Biomarkers Prev 2021;30(5): 813–21.
5. Pehlivan KC, Paul MR, Crawford JR. Central nervous system tumors in children. Pediatr Rev 2022;43(1):3–15.
6. Udaka YT, Packer RJ. Pediatric brain tumors. Neurol Clin 2018;36:533–56.
7. Lutz K, Jünger ST, Messing-Jünger M. Essential management of pediatric brain tumors. Children 2022;9(4):498.
8. Sherwen O, Baron MK, Murray NS, et al. The recognition and nursing management of common oncological emergencies in children. Br J Nurs 2022;31:20–7.
9. Ferriero DM, Fullerton HJ, Bernard TJ, et al. & American heart association stroke Council and Council on cardiovascular and stroke nursing. Management of stroke in neonates and children: a scientific statement from the American heart association/American stroke association. Stroke 2019;50(3):e51–96.
10. Lehman LL, Khoury JC, Taylor JM, et al. Pediatric stroke rates over 17 Years: report from a population-based study. J Child Neurol 2018;33(7):463–7.
11. Mallick AA, Ganesan V, Kirkham FJ, et al. Childhood arterial ischaemic stroke incidence, presenting features, and risk factors: a prospective population-based study. Lancet Neurol 2014;13(1):35–43.
12. Rivkin MJ, Bernard TJ, Dowling MM, et al. Guidelines for urgent management of stroke in children. Pediatr Neurol 2016;56:8–17.
13. McKinney SM, Magruder JT, Abramo TJ. An update on pediatric stroke protocol. Pediatr Emerg Care 2018;34(11):810–5.
14. Bernard TJ, Rivkin MJ, Scholz K, et al. On behalf of the Thrombolysis in Pediatric Stroke Study and on behalf of the Thrombolysis in Pediatric Stroke Study. Emergence of the primary pediatric stroke center: impact of the thrombolysis in pediatric stroke center. Stroke 2014;45:2018–23.

15. Harrar DB, Benedetti GM, Jayakar A, et al. Pediatric acute stroke protocols in the United States and Canada. J Pediatr 2022;242:220–7.
16. A. Bucci, DNP, CPNP-AC (email communication, January 2023).
17. Cennamo F, Masetti R, Largo P, et al. Update on febrile neutropenia in pediatric oncological patients undergoing chemotherapy. Children 2021;8(12):1086. https://doi.org/10.3390/children8121086.
18. Lekshminarayanan A, Bhatt P, Linga VG, et al. National trends in hospitalization for fever and neutropenia in children with cancer, 2007-2014. J Pediatr 2018; 202:231–7.
19. Lehrnbecher Thomas. Treatment of fever in neutropenia in pediatric oncology patients. Curr Opin Pediatr 2019;31(1):35–40.
20. Alali M, David MZ, Danziger-Isakov LA, et al. Pediatric febrile neutropenia: change in etiology of bacteremia, empiric choice of therapy and clinical outcomes. J. Pediatr.Hematol.Oncol 2020;42(6):e445.
21. Roseland J. Improving Antibiotic timing in febrile neutropenia for pediatric oncology patients with a central line. J Pediatr Oncol Nurs 2021;38(3):185–9.
22. Flood K, Rozmus J, Skippen P, et al. Fluid overload and acute kidney injury in children with tumor lysis syndrome. Pediatr Blood Cancer 2021;68(12):e29255.
23. Russell TB, Kram DE. Tumor lysis syndrome. Peds in Review 2020;41(1):20–5.
24. Williams SM, Killeen AA. Tumor lysis syndrome. Arch Pathol Lab Med 2019; 143(3):386–93.
25. Cairo MS, Bishop M. Tumour lysis syndrome: new therapeutic strategies and classification. Br J Haematol 2004;127(1):3–11.
26. Howard SC, Jones DP, Pui C. The tumor lysis syndrome. N Engl J Med 2011; 364(19):1844–54.
27. Cheung WL, Hon KL, Fung CM, et al. Tumor lysis syndrome in childhood malignancies. Drugs Context 2020;9:2019–28.
28. Webster JS, Kaplow RB. Tumor lysis syndrome: Implications for oncology nursing practice. Semin Oncol Nurs 2021;37:151136.
29. Reschke A, Richards RM, Smith SM, et al. Development of clinical pathways to improve multidisciplinary care of high-risk pediatric oncology patients. Front Oncol 2022;12:1033993.
30. Nossair F, Schoettler P, Starr J, et al. Pediatric superior vena cava syndrome: an evidence-based systematic review of the literature. Pediatr Blood Cancer 2018; 65:e27225.
31. Aljudi A, Weinzierl E, Elkhalifa M, et al. The hematological differential diagnosis of mediastinal masses. Clin Lab Med 2021;41:389–404.
32. Malik R, Mullassery D, Kleine-Brueggeney M, et al. Anterior mediastinal masses: a multidisciplinary pathway for safe diagnostic procedures. J Pediatr Surgery 2019;54:251–4.
33. Bohm A, Campbell C, Peters C, et al. Timely diagnosis and safe procedures in children with anterior mediastinal masses (AMMs): a qualitative review of the AMM protocol at BC Children's Hospital in Vancouver BC. Pediatr Hematol Oncol 2023;40(1):51–64.
34. American Society of Hematology. Sickle cell disease. Available at: https://www.hematology.org/education/patients/anemia/sickle-cell-disease.
35. Kavanagh PL, Fasipe TA, Wun T. Sickle cell disease: a review. JAMA 2022;328(1): 57–68.
36. Sedrak A, Kondamudi NP. Sickle cell disease. StatPearls. Available at: https://www.ncbi.nlm.nih.gov/books/NBK482384/.

37. Koehl JL, Koyfman A, Hayes BD, et al. High risk and low prevalence diseases: acute chest syndrome in sickle cell disease. Am J Emerg Med 2022;58:235–44.
38. Klings ES, Steinberg MH. Acute chest syndrome of sickle cell disease: Genetics, risk factors, prognosis, and management. Expert Rev Hematol 2022;15(2): 117–25.
39. Takahashi T, Okubo Y, Handa A. Acute chest syndrome among children hospitalized with vaso-occlusive crisis: a nationwide study in the United States. Pediatr Blood Cancer 2018;65(3):e26885.

Updates and Clinical Implications of Pediatric Delirium

Lauren K. Flagg, DNP, APRN, CPNP-AC[a,b,*],
Jennifer A. Mauney, DNP, APRN, CPNP-AC[c]

KEYWORDS

- Delirium • Pediatric critical care • PICU • PCICU • Pediatrics

KEY POINTS

- Delirium in pediatric critical care is a common problem associated with increased mortality, morbidity, and increased associated costs of care.
- Utilizing validated screening tools is a foundational component of identifying pediatric delirium, recommended by multiple society guidelines and position statements.
- Priority management for pediatric delirium includes risk factor reduction and optimizing the patient's environment.
- While the volume of pediatric-specific delirium research has grown over the past decade, further research is still needed regarding management strategies and outcomes.

INTRODUCTION

Delirium, as a term, is traced back more than 2000 years, with its meaning evolving from a general label for psychiatric illness to the modern interpretation, which focuses on acute fluctuations of awareness related to physical disease.[1] Starting in 1980, this definition was introduced, including hypoactive, hyperactive, and mixed subtypes of delirium.[1] Historically, it has been a psychiatric diagnosis, with the Diagnostic and Statistical Manual of Mental Disorders, Fifth Edition (DSM-5)[2] criteria including acute, fluctuating changes to a patient's attention, awareness, and cognition because of a physical etiology. During the late twentieth century, awareness of delirium within medical communities expanded, and bedside screening tools were developed to facilitate ongoing and rapid patient assessment.

There are no financial conflicts of interest to disclose.
[a] Yale University School of Nursing, Orange, CT, USA; [b] Yale New Haven Hospital, Pediatric Critical Care, New Haven, CT, USA; [c] University of Florida College of Nursing, 1225 Center Drive, PO Box 100197, Gainesville, FL 32610, USA
* Corresponding author. Yale School of Nursing, PO Box 27399, West Haven, CT 06516-0972.
E-mail address: Lauren.Flagg@yale.edu

Crit Care Nurs Clin N Am 35 (2023) 315–325
https://doi.org/10.1016/j.cnc.2023.04.006
0899-5885/23/© 2023 Elsevier Inc. All rights reserved.

ccnursing.theclinics.com

Abbreviations	
CAPD	Cornell Assessment of Pediatric Delirium
CAM-ICU	Confusion Assessment Method - Intensive Care Unit
pCAM-ICU	Pediatric Confusion Assessment Method - Intensive Care Unit
psCAM-ICU	Preschool Confusion Assessment Method - Intensive Care Unit

Within the adult population, delirium's effects have been researched extensively since the initial bedside screening tool, the Confusion Assessment Method (CAM), was developed in 1990 and the Confusion Assessment Method for the Intensive Care Unit (CAM-ICU) became available in 2001.[3,4] Over the past 30 years, research in adult intensive care units (ICUs) has shown significant links between delirium and increased mortality, morbidity, costs of care, prolonged length of stays, and requirement of long-term care facilities.[5] In a landmark study performed in 1999,[6] the management of known risk factors, such as sleep deprivation, immobility, visual and hearing impairments, dehydration, and cognitive impairments/reorientation, significantly reduced delirium rates.

Compared with adults, pediatric delirium research is in its infancy because of the recent development of pediatric assessment tools, need for expert evaluation with psychiatry, and differing developmental and cognitive abilities in the pediatric population. The first validated bedside screening tool for children was not available until 2011 and was limited to those developmentally 5 years of age and older.[7] This was followed by two additional screening tools that facilitate the assessment of children, including varying infancy periods.[8,9] Over the past decade, the volume of pediatric-specific research has grown significantly, with data showing that children have similar adverse sequelae as adults. International point prevalence data has shown a rate of 25% delirium among critically ill children, with data varying by institution and patient population.[10] Because of the potential impact of pediatric delirium, multiple society guidelines and position statements recommend routine screening using validated tools.[11–13] Despite evidence showing its patient impact and strong recommendations for routine evaluation, a recent multicenter survey across 18 countries found that only approximately 40% to 45% of pediatric critical care units routinely screen with validated tools, and less than 30% have set guidelines or protocols.[14,15]

NATURE OF THE PROBLEM

One challenge of delirium is an incomplete understanding of the multifactorial and complex mechanisms of the pathophysiology that result in acute brain dysfunction. Research in the adult population has focused on the hypothesis that delirium is caused by transient, systemic disturbances that alter neuronal activity regulation and neurotransmitter integrity.[16,17] Disruptions of cerebral blood flow and cellular equilibrium[17,18] and circadian rhythm dysregulation, with melatonin deficiency and increased cytokine release,[16] may contribute to these alterations. Key neurotransmitters thought to influence delirium pathogenesis include imbalances in γ-aminobutyric acid and serotonin; excess dopamine, glutamate, and cortisol; and deficiencies in acetylcholine.[16,17,19] Notable conditions thought to be pathophysiologic substrates of delirium include systemic inflammation in sepsis, various pharmacologic exposures (sedatives and analgesics), and postoperative procedures.[17] In summary, the central hypothesis for delirium pathophysiology is that acute alterations in neuronal and neurotransmitter activity affect the ability for proper information integration and processing within the central nervous system, leading to various clinical presentations of delirium.[16]

PREVALENCE, EPIDEMIOLOGY, AND MORTALITY RATES

The prevalence of pediatric delirium varies widely depending on the facility, unit, hospital length of stay, and patient population, with ranges reported anywhere from 12% to 65%.[20] Multiple risk factors have been associated with delirium development, encompassing nonmodifiable and iatrogenic sources. Nonmodifiable risk factors for delirium include age younger than 2 years, baseline cognitive delays, and those with higher severity illnesses.[21–23] This poses additional challenges, because children with baseline cognitive dysfunction are more difficult to screen, and validated tools have a lower sensitivity in this patient population.[8,9,24,25] Iatrogenic risk factors for delirium development include benzodiazepine and anticholinergic usage, noninvasive and invasive mechanical ventilation, vasoactive infusions, and restraints.[21,23,26] Patients with prolonged critical care admissions of more than 2 to 5 days have shown a significantly higher delirium prevalence, and patients who were ever delirious had an initial delirium diagnosis more frequently made within the first 72 hours of ICU admission.[10,20,21] Generally, pediatric ICUs (PICUs) have a slightly lower prevalence, commonly reporting ranges averaging 20% to 30%.[10,20,23] Conversely, pediatric cardiac ICUs (PCICUs) observe higher rates, often reporting prevalence rates of 40% to 50%.[20,26,27] This may be attributed to increased risk factors in PCICU patients, such as cardiopulmonary bypass, vasoactive infusions, and mechanical ventilation.[23,27]

The effect of delirium on patient outcomes is also significant, with negative impacts on pediatric mortality and morbidity. An overall 85% increase in critical care costs has been found in pediatric delirium.[28] As with adult data, delirium has been found to be an independent predictor of mortality, with hospital mortality significantly increasing after controlling for illness severity.[21] In addition to increased mortality, delirious children have increased morbidity with prolonged days of mechanical ventilation, ICU and hospital length of stay, ICU readmission rates, and cognitive decline.[21–23,27,28] Furthermore, post-ICU syndrome and posttraumatic stress complications of pediatric critical care have begun to be linked to possible prior delirium in small studies.[29,30] Recent literature also supports a link between decreased quality of life following PICU or PCICU discharge in patients that had been delirious during their stay.[31,32]

EVALUATION

The first validated bedside screening tool for children developmentally 5 years of age and older, the pediatric CAM-ICU (pCAM-ICU), was initially published in 2011.[7] This was followed by the Cornell Assessment of Pediatric Delirium (CAP-D) in 2014[8] and preschool CAM-ICU (psCAM-ICU) in 2016,[9] expanding the assessment to newborns and children as young as 6 months of age, respectively. More recently, in 2021, the psCAM included validation for children younger than 6 months of age.[33]

Although these tools allow bedside assessment of delirium in critically ill pediatric patients, there are fundamental differences in how and when they are performed. The pCAM-ICU and psCAM-ICU evaluate using DSM-5 criteria for delirium diagnosis versus the CAP-D, which serves as a screening tool only, requiring further investigation to make an official diagnosis.[7,8,24] Scheduled screening for the CAP-D and p/psCAM-ICU occurs every shift (twice daily),[7–9] whereas the p/psCAM-ICU may also be performed as needed to reflect additional mentation or level of consciousness disruptions.[7,9] Conversely, the CAP-D is an assessment reflective of a more extended period of cumulative time, so it is recommended to be performed in the last several hours of a nurse's shift.[8]

There is only one study[24] that directly compares the accuracy of the CAP-D and psCAM/pCAM-ICU tools to DSM-5 diagnostic criteria, allowing the evaluation of variables during routine PICU care that may affect their accuracy. This study found performance variability in all screening tools, with the CAP-D having higher sensitivity (91.3%) than the ps/pCAM-ICU (58.8% and 75%).[24] However, the CAP-D had a lower specificity (CAP-D, 75.2%; psCAM-ICU, 89.8%; pCAM-ICU, 84.9%).[24] Specific factors identified as leading to CAP-D and psCAM-ICU incongruity with the DSM-5 included younger age and receiving of sedation.[24]

The Pediatric and Preschool Confusion Assessment Method for the Intensive Care Unit

The pCAM-ICU[7] was the first validated pediatric delirium assessment tool, introduced in 2011 and based on the well-established CAM and CAM-ICU adult tools. This tool focused on children with a cognition level at or higher than a with a Richmond Agitation Sedation Scale of −3 or higher (responsive to verbal stimulation).[7] Following the creation of the pCAM-ICU, the psCAM-ICU[9] was created to assess pediatric patients younger than 5 years of age. Initial inclusion criteria were limited to children 6 months to 5 years of age, excluding children with hearing or visual impairments, severe cognitive delays, non-English speaking, or those receiving end-of-life care.[9] Recently, this age range was expanded to include children younger than 6 months old.[33] The p/psCAM-ICU focus on assessing four primary features of delirium: (1) acute or fluctuating mental examination changes, (2) inattention, (3) altered level of consciousness, and (4) disorganized thinking.[7,9]

To diagnose delirium, a positive p/psCAM-ICU requires the identification of abnormal behaviors in features one and two, in addition to features three or four.[7,9] The first feature assesses for change in the patient's mental status from baseline or fluctuations over the past 24 hours.[7,9] The second feature assesses for inattention, with the pCAM-ICU[7] using a sequence of simple commands and the psCAM-ICU[9] using picture and mirror cards combined with verbal prompting. If either of the first two assessment points is normal, the screener is prompted to stop screening because delirium is precluded.[7,9] For all age ranges, the third feature identifies an altered level of consciousness using Richmond Agitation Sedation Scale scoring, with any number other than "0" (awake and calm) identifying delirium presence.[7,9] Feature four evaluates disorganized thinking and is performed only if there is no change in the level of consciousness noted in feature three.[7,9] In children developmentally older than 5 years of age, this section consists of a series of five predefined questions and simple commands. Disorganized thinking is considered present if the patient cannot complete four items correctly.[7] In children younger than 5 years of age developmentally, this section focuses on assessing sleep-wake cycle disturbances.[9]

The Cornell Assessment of Pediatric Delirium

The CAP-D was created as a rapid observational screening tool and was an adaption of the Pediatric Anesthesia Emergence Delirium tool, which had the limitation of identifying only the subtype of hyperactive delirium.[8] The CAP-D was validated in 2014 by assessing the tool in conjunction with an independent psychiatrist evaluation of PICU patients from birth to 21 years of age.[8] This tool comprises eight questions, each on a five-point Likert-type scale, allowing a total cumulative score of up to 32.[8] The best specificity and sensitivity to delirium detection was found at a score of nine or higher.[8]

Key components of this tool include its comprehensive, scaled screening, ability to capture varying presentations of delirium, twice-daily cumulative scoring by the bedside nurse, and incorporation of developmentally informed observations.[8] The developmental anchor points provide context for age-appropriate behaviors of newborns to 2 years old while being assessed by the CAP-D tool.[34] The use of this additional supplement to the CAP-D screening tool allows for a more reliable, age-specific screening of delirium by various providers and addresses the complexity of evaluating the cognition and consciousness of infants. Lastly, evaluation of the CAP-D screening tool highlights the challenge of diagnosing delirium in the cognitively delayed pediatric population. However, although it has an increased rate of false positives, it is still noted to demonstrate applicability in this population.[8] Future implications have focused on the recommendation for inclusion of baseline (before acute illness) scoring and potential scoring adjustment to account for these baseline developmental domains.[8,25,34]

GUIDELINES

With the significant concern for the potential impact of pediatric delirium, society guidelines, clinical pathways, and position statements have recently provided consensus recommendations for pediatric delirium, including assessment, screening tools, and nonpharmacologic and pharmacologic strategies.[11–13] In 2016, the European Society of Paediatric and Neonatal Intensive Care published a position statement for health care professionals. For this statement, a group of multidisciplinary experts provided clinical recommendations on assessing delirium, withdrawal, pain, and level of distress and sedation through a literature review of assessment tools' psychometric properties and group consensus.[11] The development of a clinical practice pathway was later published in the American Academy of Pediatrics (2019) following a literature review and consensus by an international workgroup of pediatric psychiatry experts.[12] This clinical practice pathway, divided into a two-part flowchart of prevention and identification, and diagnosis and management, provides overall guidance on physiologic, pharmacologic, and environmental factors within the preventative measures, work-up, and treatment of hospital inpatient pediatric delirium.[12]

In 2022, the Society of Critical Care Medicine published the "Clinical Practice Guidelines on Prevention and Management of Pain, Agitation, Neuromuscular Blockade, and Delirium in Critically Ill Pediatric Patients With Consideration of the ICU Environment and Early Mobility" following a 12-year taskforce initiative consisting of literature and quality of evidence review, and the development of key recommendations and good practice statements.[13]

A significant recommendation from these guidelines is using validated and reliable delirium screening tools.[11–13] These validated tools are identified as either the CAP-D[11–13] or p/psCAM-ICU.[12,13] Furthermore, the importance of scheduled routine screening of critically ill pediatric patients is emphasized by European Society of Paediatric and Neonatal Intensive Care and Society of Critical Care Medicine.[11,13] Evaluation of environmental sources and iatrogenic factors that may pose a risk of delirium development is also recommended.[11,12] Pharmacologic management of severe and clinically significant delirium symptoms with antipsychotics or sedation adjuncts is addressed.[11–13] Lastly, a multidisciplinary approach and expert consultation for pediatric delirium is highlighted.[6,12]

COMMON BARRIERS TO SCREENING AND STRATEGIES

Within the pediatric critical care population, delirium research continues to expand the identification of barriers to screening implementation, accuracy, and sustainability. Common barriers identified include nurse hesitation, workflow interruptions, inconsistent documentation, inadequate education or familiarity with the tool, and difficulties incorporating delirium screening in electronic medical records.[35–37] Further barriers identified in the literature include heavy workload, lack of understanding of tool utilization with sedated patients or those with cognitive delays, and concern for an inconsistent medical approach to positive delirium screen.[35]

A multifaceted approach is vital to addressing barriers to screening. Addressing these barriers has centered on the importance of nursing education on pediatric delirium and the improved perception of the direct impact of delirium screening protocols on improved patient care.[35] Although delirium screening compliance may increase following initial nurse education, sustainability requires ongoing support, such as additional training, nursing champions, screening reminders, and tool/protocol integration into the electronic medical record.[35,37]

THERAPEUTIC OPTIONS

Approaches to delirium prevention and management have advanced from a combination of mitigating established delirium risk factors and extrapolation from adult research. Nonpharmacologic and pharmacologic strategies address the multicomponent physiologic and environmental elements associated with pediatric delirium.

Nonpharmacologic

Inouye and colleagues[6] found that providing a collective group of cognitive, environmental, and physiologic interventions helped to reduce delirium in adults. This program has formed a standard for delirium reduction models emphasizing the normalization of day-to-day routines and mimicking baseline functional level activities as much as possible.[38] Although much of the available data are from adult populations, recent pediatric-specific research on the efficacy of nonpharmacologic delirium reduction bundles has shown significant delirium reductions in children less than 5 years of age and those post congenital heart surgery.[39]

Physiologic delirium prevention and management strategies focus on nutrition, elimination, sleep, and mobility.[12] Ensuring adequate hydration and nutrition are central to health promotion and healing.[6] Initial delirium prevention measures include normalizing bodily functions by promoting regular bowel and bladder elimination and minimizing lines and tubes.[12] Promoting mobilization and clinically, developmentally appropriate activities are also integral to physiologic improvements.[6,12] Although pediatric-specific data on early mobility and patient outcomes are developing, what is available thus far has shown low rates of adverse events and is supported for inclusion in patient care guidelines from national and international medical societies.[11–13,40]

Environmental and cognitive strategies focus on techniques that prioritize sleep hygiene, optimize cognition, and encourage familiarity within unfamiliar environments.[12] Noise, light pollution, and frequent interruptions, such as vital signs, assessments, and interventions, disrupt good sleep hygiene in the ICU.[6,12] Optimizing day and night routines help support the prevention and management of delirium.[6,12] Simple actions, such as reorientation, using patient names, consistently introducing care team members, and using developmentally appropriate language, can support cognitive function and orientation.[6,12] Addressing the immediate environment by including familiar, comfort items from home, and encouraging family involvement with patient care, are environmental strategies that contribute to normalizing the unfamiliar critical care environment.[12]

With any concern for delirium, it is essential to evaluate for underlying cause or contributing factors. Although the critical care environment, illness severity, and unfamiliar surroundings may all contribute significantly to delirium development, it remains imperative to identify any new physiologic changes that may have led to the awareness or cognition change.[38] There are several mnemonics available to help guide

Table 1
Evaluation mnemonic for modifiable pediatric delirium contributors

Mnemonic	Assessment/Intervention
Bring oxygen	Evaluate for hypoxia, decreased cardiac output, anemia
Remove/reduce	Reduce/avoid anticholinergics, benzodiazepines, high-dose opioids
Atmosphere	Assess noise/light levels, reorient, encourage family involvement, avoid restraints
Infection/inflammation/ immobilization	Assess for new infection or inflammatory process, evaluate ability to mobilize
New organ dysfunction	Consider all body systems (including central nervous system), assess renal and liver function
Metabolic disturbance	Evaluate for electrolyte derangements, acid/base status
Awake	Assess for sleep/wake cycle disruption
Pain	Evaluate for undertreated/overtreated, optimize nonopiates, nonpharmacologic strategies
Sedation	Avoid under/over sedation, set daily sedation goals, use dexmedetomidine in place of benzodiazepine

Based on Information from Smith et al (2013)[40] and Bettencourt and Mullen (2017).[18]

this evaluation, such as the commonly cited "BRAINMAPS" (**Table 1**), developed by Smith and colleagues[40] This mnemonic includes possible environmental, pharmacologic, and physiologic causes, such as hypoxemia, decreased cardiac output, metabolic derangements, and organ dysfunction.[40]

Pharmacologic

There are limited data on the pharmacologic treatment of pediatric delirium. Additionally, there are no proven pharmacologic treatments for delirium in the adult or pediatric populations.[13,19] Society guideline consensus and additional literature focus on pharmacologic management that prioritizes treatment of underlying medical conditions and iatrogenic factors.[11–13,19] These considerations include physiologic dysfunction, polypharmacy, benzodiazepine exposure, and iatrogenic withdrawal syndrome.[11–13]

The primary consensus for pharmacologic intervention is to minimize overall sedation and to limit, reduce, or avoid benzodiazepine exposure.[11–13] Within the adult population, benzodiazepine-sparing sedation regimens with the adjunct of dexmedetomidine has been found to decrease delirium occurrence.[41] Furthermore, in a large randomized control trial, a reduction in the duration of delirium has not been found in the adult population receiving antipsychotics.[42] Routine pharmacologic treatment with antipsychotic drugs is not recommended and is reserved for refractory or severe delirium.[13,19]

Limited data have noted the off-label use of antipsychotics in children, such as haloperidol, quetiapine, or risperidone, to show benefit in delirium screens.[11,19,43,44] When using antipsychotic therapies in pediatric delirium, consideration should be given to reducing total drug exposure and limiting administration to severe or refractory delirium symptoms. It must be balanced with the significant safety concerns of possible adverse effects, such as cardiac or hepatic dysfunctions.[13,43] Because data on efficacy and long-term effects are limited, the use of antipsychotics is not currently approved by the US Food and Drug Administration for delirium management in the pediatric population.[13] Further research is needed to guide the use of antipsychotic medications in severe pediatric delirium.

FUTURE DIRECTIONS

As clinical awareness has expanded, current literature and professional societies recommend routine delirium screening and the expansion of pediatric delirium research. Future research directions may take several avenues, including methods for optimizing screening tools, management guidelines, and patient outcomes. Evaluation of outcomes and the impact of prevention and management strategies are contingent on the ability to have consistent and global delirium screening, resulting in large-scale patient populations.

Despite the increased breadth of pediatric-specific research, clinical decision-making continues to rely on foundations within adult data because of the overall suboptimal pediatric screening rates. Additionally, the inpatient pediatric population is unique because of the range of developmental levels. Although strides have been made to better address the specificity of screening tools in young (<2 years of age) patients and those with cognitive impairments, these populations are at a higher risk of developing delirium and are more challenging to screen accurately.[8,10,19,25] Future implications may focus on the recommendation to consider a child's baseline delirium score/developmental level and allow for scoring adjustments.[8,34] Another possibility includes combining delirium and agitation/sedation scoring tools within a single assessment tool and granting the potential to differentiate delirium subtypes.

Regarding patient outcomes, post-ICU syndrome and trauma related to ICU care have been well described. Research before the advent of bedside screening tools links pediatric patients who reported hallucinations while admitted to the ICU as having higher posttraumatic stress scores.[30] With improvements in delirium screening, there have been hypothesized connections to delirium and posttraumatic stress disorder after discharge in pediatric patients.[45] Other research has begun to explore the quality of life scores and the associated implications in pediatric critical care delirium.[32]

SUMMARY

Delirium in critically ill children is a concerning condition associated with increased mortality and morbidity. Despite these deleterious effects, delirium remains underrecognized because of suboptimal screening and protocol implementation in pediatric critical care units nationally and internationally. As a result of suboptimal screening practices and overall lower frequency of critically ill pediatric patients compared with adults, pediatric-specific delirium research in prevention and management has lagged comparatively. There remains a strong need for high-quality evidence to affect clinical prevalence and guide future nonpharmacologic and pharmacologic pediatric delirium management.

CLINICS CARE POINTS

- Routine delirium screening with validated tools in pediatric critical care units remains suboptimal, despite recommendations by multiple society guidelines.
- Patients with cognitive dysfunction have increased risk of becoming delirious and present challenges to assessment due to lower tool sensitivity and specificity.
- The mainstay of pediatric delirium prevention and management is non-pharmacologic, focusing on condition identification, screening tool use, and normalizing a patient's environment.

- With any concern for delirium, it is vital to evaluate for a new underlying physiologic change and reduce or eliminate other potential contributing factors.
- Some pharmacologic strategies exist for both delirium prevention and severe symptom management, though research is limited regarding the use of antipsychotics in delirious children.

REFERENCES

1. Deksnytė A, Aranauskas R, Budrys V, et al. Delirium: its historical evolution and current interpretation. Eur J Intern Med 2012;23(6):483–6.
2. European Delirium Association; American Delirium Society. The DSM-5 criteria, level of arousal and delirium diagnosis: inclusiveness is safer. BMC Med 2014; 12:141.
3. Ely EW, Margolin R, Francis J, et al. Evaluation of delirium in critically ill patients: validation of the Confusion Assessment Method for the Intensive Care Unit (CAM-ICU). Crit Care Med 2001;29(7):1370–9.
4. Inouye SK, van Dyck CH, Alessi CA, et al. Clarifying confusion: the Confusion Assessment Method. A new method for detection of delirium. Ann Intern Med 1990;113(12):941–8.
5. Salluh JI, Wang H, Schneider EB, et al. Outcome of delirium in critically ill patients: systematic review and meta-analysis. BMJ 2015;350:h2538.
6. Inouye SK, Bogardus ST Jr, Charpentier PA, et al. A multicomponent intervention to prevent delirium in hospitalized older patients. N Engl J Med 1999;340(9):669–76.
7. Smith HA, Boyd J, Fuchs DC, et al. Diagnosing delirium in critically ill children: validity and reliability of the pediatric Confusion Assessment Method for the intensive care unit. Crit Care Med 2011;39(1):150–7.
8. Traube C, Silver G, Kearney J, et al. Cornell Assessment of Pediatric Delirium: a valid, rapid, observational tool for screening delirium in the PICU. Crit Care Med 2014;42(3):656–63.
9. Smith HA, Gangopadhyay M, Goben CM, et al. The preschool Confusion Assessment Method for the ICU: valid and reliable delirium monitoring for critically ill infants and children. Crit Care Med 2016;44(3):592–600.
10. Traube C, Silver G, Reeder RW, et al. Delirium in critically ill children: an international point prevalence study. Crit Care Med 2017;45(4):584–90.
11. Harris J, Ramelet AS, van Dijk M, et al. Clinical recommendations for pain, sedation, withdrawal and delirium assessment in critically ill infants and children: an ESPNIC position statement for healthcare professionals. Intensive Care Med 2016;42(6):972–86.
12. Silver GH, Kearney JA, Bora S, et al. A clinical pathway to standardize care of children with delirium in pediatric inpatient settings. Hosp Pediatr 2019;9(11): 909–16.
13. Smith HAB, Besunder JB, Betters KA, et al. 2022 Society of Critical Care Medicine clinical practice guidelines on prevention and management of pain, agitation, neuromuscular blockade, and delirium in critically ill pediatric patients with consideration of the ICU environment and early mobility. Pediatr Crit Care Med 2022;23(2):e74–110.
14. Ista E, Redivo J, Kananur P, et al. ABCDEF bundle practices for critically ill children: an international survey of 161 PICUs in 18 countries. Crit Care Med 2022; 50(1):114–25.

15. Valentine K, Cisco MJ, Lasa JJ, et al. A survey of current practices in sedation, analgesia, withdrawal, and delirium management in paediatric cardiac ICUs. Cardiol Young 2023;1–6. https://doi.org/10.1017/S1047951122004115, published online ahead of print, 2023 Jan 10.

16. Maldonado JR. Delirium pathophysiology: an updated hypothesis of the etiology of acute brain failure. Int J Geriatr Psychiatry 2018;33(11):1428–57.

17. Gunther ML, Morandi A, Ely EW. Pathophysiology of delirium in the intensive care unit. Crit Care Clin 2008;24(1):45–viii.

18. Bettencourt A, Mullen JE. Delirium in children: identification, prevention, and management. Crit Care Nurse 2017;37(3):e9–18.

19. Siegel E, Traube C. Pediatric delirium: epidemiology and outcomes. Curr Opin Pediatr 2020;32(6):743–9.

20. Patel AK, Bell MJ, Traube C. Delirium in pediatric critical care. Pediatr Clin North Am 2017;64(5):1117–32.

21. Traube C, Silver G, Gerber LM, et al. Delirium and mortality in critically ill children: epidemiology and outcomes of pediatric delirium. Crit Care Med 2017;45(5):891–8.

22. Pilato TC, Mauer EA, Gerber LM, et al. Pediatric delirium and all-cause PICU readmissions within 1 year. Pediatr Crit Care Med 2022;23(10):766–73.

23. Dervan LA, Di Gennaro JL, Farris RWD, et al. Delirium in a tertiary PICU: risk factors and outcomes. Pediatr Crit Care Med 2020;21(1):21–32.

24. Paterson RS, Kenardy JA, Dow BL, et al. Accuracy of delirium assessments in critically ill children: a prospective, observational study during routine care. Aust Crit Care 2021;34(3):226–34.

25. Kaur S, Silver G, Samuels S, et al. Delirium and developmental disability: improving specificity of a pediatric delirium screen. Pediatr Crit Care Med 2020;21(5):409–14.

26. Staveski SL, Pickier RH, Khoury PR, et al. Prevalence of ICU delirium in postoperative pediatric cardiac surgery patients. Pediatr Crit Care Med 2021;22:68–78.

27. Alvarez RV, Palmer C, Czaja AS, et al. Delirium is a common and early finding in patients in the pediatric cardiac intensive care unit. J Pediatr 2018;195:206–12.

28. Traube C, Mauer EA, Gerber LM, et al. Cost associated with pediatric delirium in the ICU. Crit Care Med 2016;44(12):e1175–9.

29. Traube C. Beware the aftermath: delirium and post-intensive care syndrome in critically ill children. Pediatr Crit Care Med 2022;23(2):144–6.

30. Colville G, Kerry S, Pierce C. Children's factual and delusional memories of intensive care. Am J Respir Crit Care Med 2008;177(9):976–82.

31. Silver G, Doyle H, Hegel E, et al. Association between pediatric delirium and quality of life after discharge. Crit Care Med 2020;48(12):1829–34.

32. Dervan LA, Killien EY, Smith MB, et al. Health-related quality of life following delirium in the PICU. Pediatr Crit Care Med 2022;23(2):118–28.

33. Canter MO, Tanguturi YC, Ellen Wilson J, et al. Prospective validation of the preschool Confusion Assessment Method for the ICU to screen for delirium in infants less than 6 months old. Crit Care Med 2021;49(10):e902–9.

34. Silver G, Kearney J, Traube C, et al. Delirium screening anchored in child development: the Cornell Assessment for Pediatric Delirium. Palliat Support Care 2015;13(4):1005–11.

35. Mallick N, Mize M, Patel AK. Implementation of a pediatric delirium screening program in a pediatric intensive care unit. Crit Care Nurse 2022;42(3):37–45.

36. Franken A, Sebbens D, Mensik J. Pediatric delirium: early identification of barriers to optimize success of screening and prevention. J Pediatr Health Care 2019; 33(3):228–33.
37. Eken HN, Betters KA, Fuchs DC, et al. Improving delirium assessments in Vanderbilt pediatric and pediatric cardiovascular intensive care units. Pediatric Quality & Safety 2022;7(4):e577.
38. Hshieh TT, Yang T, Gartaganis SL, et al. Hospital elder life program: systematic review and meta-analysis of effectiveness. Am J Geriatr Psychiatry 2018; 26(10):1015–33.
39. Michel J, Schepan E, Hofbeck M, et al. Implementation of a delirium bundle for pediatric intensive care patients. Front Pediatr 2022;10:826259.
40. Smith HA, Brink E, Fuchs DC, et al. Pediatric delirium: monitoring and management in the pediatric intensive care unit. Pediatr Clin North Am 2013;60(3): 741–60.
41. Burry LD, Cheng W, Williamson DR, et al. Pharmacological and non-pharmacological interventions to prevent delirium in critically ill patients: a systematic review and network meta-analysis. Intensive Care Med 2021;47(9): 943–60.
42. Girard TD, Exline MC, Carson SS, et al. Haloperidol and ziprasidone for treatment of delirium in critical illness. N Engl J Med 2018;379(26):2506–16.
43. Turkel SB, Hanft A. The pharmacologic management of delirium in children and adolescents. Paediatr Drugs 2014;16(4):267–74.
44. Thielen JR, Sawyer JE, Henry BM, et al. Short-term effect of quetiapine used to treat delirium symptoms on opioid and benzodiazepine requirements in the pediatric cardiac intensive care unit. Pediatr Cardiol 2022. https://doi.org/10.1007/s00246-022-02980-3.
45. Turkel SB. Pediatric delirium: recognition, management, and outcome. Curr Psychiatry Rep 2017;19(12):101.

Nurse-Led Rounds in the Pediatric Intensive Care Unit

Lindsey Bird, DNP, APN, CPNP-AC, CNE[a,b],
Vanessa Kalis, DNP, CPNP-AC, ACNP, CNS, CHSE, FAANP[c],
Leah Apalodimas, MSN, APN, CCRN, CPNP-AC/PC[a,b],*

KEYWORDS

- Pediatric intensive care unit (PICU) • Cardiac intensive care unit (CICU)
- Multidisciplinary rounds • Nurse-led rounds

KEY POINTS

- Interprofessional communication and collaboration are imperative to patient safety and quality outcomes.
- Multidisciplinary rounds are a mainstay of team communication, but their use does not ensure desired outcomes in the absence of appropriate team member engagement.
- Nursing participation in rounds is imperative, but workflow variations often inhibit their presence.
- Nurse-led rounds ensure nursing presence and confer additional patient and staff benefits, but there is a very small amount of data about implementation of this process.
- Nurse-led rounds have been successfully implemented in 4 diverse pediatric critical care service lines with positive outcomes in multiple domains.

INTRODUCTION

The pediatric intensive care unit (PICU) is a dynamic, complex environment with high propensity for medical error.[1-4] Numerous studies support that the greatest risks for error are team communication and collaboration failures.[1-8] To mitigate these risks and enhance patient outcomes, many PICUs use multidisciplinary bedside rounds as the foundation of their workflow.[5,9-12] Although the bedside nurse has a unique patient perspective, their role in bedside rounds has been heterogeneous, and their ability to participate has been inconsistent.[13-16] Lack of bedside nursing engagement in rounds compromises the safeguards that rounds are meant to establish.[9-16] In

[a] College of Nursing, University of Tennessee Health Science Center, 874 Union Avenue, Memphis, TN 38103, USA; [b] Division of Pediatric Cardiollgy, Le Bonheur Children's Hospital, 51 North Dunlap Street, Memphis, TN 38103, USA; [c] Division of Critical Care, Children's Hospital of Orange County, 1201 W La Veta Avenue, Orange, CA 92868, USA
* Corresponding author. Le Bonheur Children's Hospital, The Heart Institute, 3rd Floor, 51 North Dunlap Street, Memphis, TN 38103.
E-mail address: lapalodi@uthsc.edu

Crit Care Nurs Clin N Am 35 (2023) 327–336
https://doi.org/10.1016/j.cnc.2023.05.013
0899-5885/23/© 2023 Elsevier Inc. All rights reserved.

acknowledging barriers to nurse participation in rounds, some institutions have shifted from provider-led to nurse-led rounds and have shared diverse experiences and outcomes.[17,18]

BACKGROUND

Literature has well described the necessity of bedside multidisciplinary rounds for information sharing, shared decision making, and team collaboration.[1,4–6,8–10,19,20] These tenets directly benefit patients via reduced morbidity, mortality, and length of stay; furthermore, benefits extend to staff via enhanced feelings of value and mutual respect.[5,19–22] This knowledge, however, has not eliminated obstacles to bedside nurse engagement in rounds.[4,5,8,9,13] Team failure to coordinate timing with nurses, conflict with nursing workflow, and overall time spent per patient reduce the likelihood of nurse attendance and participation.[5,8,13] The transition from provider to nurse-led rounds addresses these barriers by restructuring the rounding framework around nurses themselves. Despite the breadth of data on the importance of nursing engagement in rounds, few support this specific model or the barriers in adopting it.[17,18] The available body of literature supports that nurse-led rounds not only generate interdisciplinary collaboration and positive clinical sequelae but also increase nurse and family satisfaction.[14,17,18,21] These findings are of particular interest given the relationship between nursing job satisfaction and intent to leave or remain in the profession.[11,17,23] The interconnectedness of team communication, job satisfaction, and patient outcomes prompted 4 pediatric critical care service lines to implement nurse-led multidisciplinary rounds. Their experiences and outcomes are detailed in later discussion.

DISCUSSION
Le Bonheur Children's Hospital Experience

Le Bonheur Children's Hospital in Memphis, Tennessee is a 255-bed pediatric teaching hospital associated with the University of Tennessee Health Science Center. Nurse-led rounds have been instituted within 3 different critical care units for the purposes of improving bedside nurse engagement, promoting bedside teaching with the multidisciplinary team (not exclusive to providers only), ensuring clear and closed-loop communication regarding the daily medical plan among the multidisciplinary team, and promoting bedside nurse professional development.

Intermediate care unit

The Intermediate Care Unit (IMCU) is a 12-bed step-down unit overseen daily by a dedicated team of critical care advanced practice nurses (APNs) and an attending physician. This was the first unit to implement nurse-led rounds at Le Bonheur Children's Hospital in 2014. The APNs led the initiative, with strong attending physician support from the Critical Care medical division. The first draft of the rounding tool was developed by the APNs and was structured to include acute events or significant clinical status changes from the previous 12 hours, the nurse's physical assessment of the patient organized by systems, and the current medical plan. Following the nurse's presentation, the APN formulates the medical plan along with the attending physician and leads bedside teaching for the team. At the completion of rounds for the patient, the bedside nurse summarizes the plan to ensure closed-loop communication.

To promote team buy-in and adoption of the tool, a work group, including a lead APN, 2 charge nurses, a unit-based nurse manager, and the IMCU nursing director, was convened. The initial tool was presented to the work group and went through several iterations. The nurses preferred a tool that would also support hand-off of patients at shift change. Thus, the tool includes some information presented in a way that is more conducive to nursing hand-off than a rounding presentation of a medical plan. The APNs agreed that for ease of use and increased probability that the tool would be used, it would be acceptable to include some of the key nursing information that was requested (eg, drug allergies or gastrostomy tube size). The IMCU rounding

Intermediate Care Unit Rounding Tool

Name/Label:	Age _____ **Check Fridge Temp**
	Code Status _____
	Head Circumference _____ qMon Monthly
	Weight:_____ Daily MonThu MonThuSat
Problem List:	Reason For Current Admission:
	Isolation/Precautions:
	Neuro
Allergies:	WAT:_____
	Wean:
Respiratory: .... VAP	Pain _____
	Tmax:_____
RR____ PIP or TV/PEEP___/____ PS____ FiO2____	Therapies: PT / OT / ST
O2 Sats_____	CAP-D Score_____
RR:____	CHEER Level_____
	Cardiac .... VTE Risk
	HR:_____ BP:_____
Breath Sounds/WOB .... Trach ▲	VTE Prophylaxis_____
GI/GU: .... CAUTI	IVF/CVAD/Infusions .... CLABSI
Fluid Balance: _____	Type of line_____
UOP/Stool Output: _____cc/kg/hr	
Last BM_____	
Foley:	Dressing ▲ _____ Cap ▲ _____ Tubing ▲ _____
Diet/Feeds	Musculoskeletal/Skin: ...... Pressure Injury
Equipment: (drains, SCDs, etc.)	Activity Level: OOB ...... Braden/Braden Q Score ____
	Surgeries/Procedures/Tests/labs in last 24 hrs:
New orders/Misc:	Social/Trach training
	Skill .... Caregiver 1 Caregiver 2
	Suctioning _____ _____
Current concerns and Anticipated Concerns	Trach care _____ _____
	Trach Change _____ _____
	CPR _____ _____
Short Term Goal	Long Term Goal
	Reviewed 01/24/2023

Fig. 1. IMCU rounding tool. Nursing presentation rounding tool for the IMCU at Le Bonheur Children's Hospital in Memphis, Tennessee.

tool (**Fig. 1**) is viewed as a living document by the team and is adjusted as needed by both nurses and providers.

Implementation of nurse-led rounds in the IMCU was met with some unforeseen challenges. Most notably, nurses were not accustomed to the style of teaching that is prominent on traditional medical rounds. Knowledge-seeking questions from providers were perceived by the nurses as intimidating and challenging. Although the medical providers experienced the interaction as an active discussion, the nurses felt that they were under an interrogation. Very quickly, trust and collegiality between the nurses, APNs, and physicians broke down owing to the drastic culture change that accompanied nurse-led rounds.

A couple of strategies were used to remedy the relationship breakdown between the nurses and medical providers. First, half-day retreats were organized with small groups of nurses and 1 to 2 medical providers at a time. The retreats were led by the hospital chaplain so that moderation of discussion was led by a neutral individual. Following the retreats, a short series of meetings with the initial work group were held to provide periodic check points and feedback on the state of the new rounding culture. In addition, the medical providers modified their teaching style to include a mini-lecture on pertinent disease processes or relevant medical literature. Discussion and questions were purposefully generated between the APNs and physicians to role model and normalize this type of interaction. Nurses were present for the teaching and encouraged to ask questions to glean a deeper comprehension but were never asked questions in return by the medical providers. After completing the retreats and a few months of using the new teaching techniques, the relationships were repaired. Even more importantly, nurse-led rounds were successfully adopted into the culture of the unit, and there was a clearly appreciated improvement in the nurses' understanding of their patients' pathophysiology and medical plan.

Extracorporeal membrane oxygenation service line

The PICU at Le Bonheur Children's Hospital, like many PICUs in teaching hospitals throughout the United States, is staffed primarily with resident physicians as front-line providers. The resident learning supportive culture was a barrier to implementing nurse-led rounds within the entire unit. However, the extracorporeal membrane oxygenation (ECMO) patient population presented an opportunity to leverage nursing engagement during rounds, particularly because clear and collaborative communication is essential among the interdisciplinary teams involved with these patients.

The ECMO team consists of ECMO specialists, which are composed of 38 critical care nurses and 2 critical care respiratory therapists, a medical director, and 4 critical care physicians who support ECMO services outside of their regular PICU service. ECMO patients are cared for in the PICU and Cardiac Intensive Care Unit (CICU) at Le Bonheur Children's Hospital. Neonatal patients requiring ECMO support are transferred to the PICU for their care. This arrangement makes care of ECMO patients inherently complex. Multiple disciplines (eg, neonatology, cardiothoracic surgery, general surgery, infectious disease, nephrology) frequently consult and offer recommendations. The ECMO service line assimilates this input to streamline care and bridge the gap between consultants and the primary service line. Nevertheless, the ECMO specialists found that even with this model, large disparities existed in daily management goals for these patients, often creating confusion for the specialist and bedside nurse.

ECMO specialist-led rounds were created to address the problem of unclear management goals. The initiative was led by 2 senior nurses on the ECMO specialist team. The rounding tool (**Fig. 2**) was specially designed to promote presentation of

Extracorporeal Membrane Oxygenation Service Line Rounding Tool

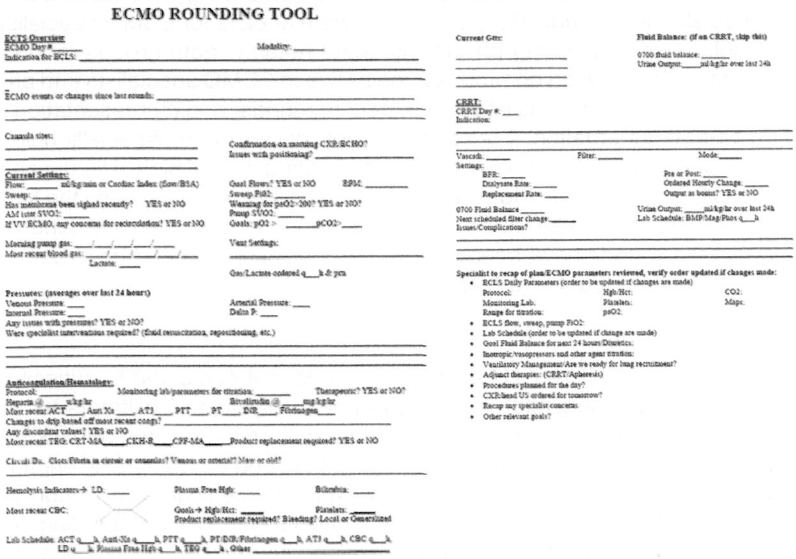

ECMO ROUNDING TOOL

ECTS Overview:
ECMO Day #____ Modality: ____
Indication for ECLS: ____

ECMO events or changes since last rounds: ____

Cannula sites: ____
Confirmation on morning CXR/ECHO?
Issues with positioning? ____

Current Settings:
Flow: ____ ml/kg/min or Cardiac Index (flow/BSA)
Sweep: ____
Has membrane been sighed recently? YES or NO
AM tmt SVO2: ____
If VV ECMO, any concerns for recirculation? YES or NO
Goal Flows? YES or NO RPM: ____
Sweep FiO2: ____
Weaning for paO2>200? YES or NO?
Pump SVO2: ____
Goals: pO2 > ____ pCO2> ____

Morning pump gas: ____/____/____/____/____
Most recent blood gas: ____/____/____/____/____
Lactate: ____
Vent Settings: ____
Gas/Lactate ordered q___h & prn

Pressures: (averages over last 24 hours)
Venous Pressure: ____
Internal Pressure: ____
Arterial Pressure: ____
Delta P: ____
Any issues with pressures? YES or NO?
Were specialist interventions required? (fluid resuscitation, repositioning, etc.)

Anticoagulation/Hematology:
Protocol: ____ Monitoring lab/parameters for titration: ____ Therapeutic? YES or NO?
Heparin @ ____ u/kg/hr Bivalirudin @ ____ mg/kg/hr
Most recent ACT____, Anti Xa ____, AT3____, PTT____, PT____, INR____, Fibrinogen____
Changes to drip based off most recent coags? ____
Any discordant values? YES or NO
Most recent TEG: CRT-MA____ CKH-R____ CFF-MA____ Product replacement required? YES or NO

Circuit Dx. Clots/Fibrin in circuit or cannulas? Venous or arterial? New or old?

Hemolysis Indicators→ LD: ____ Plasma Free Hgb: ____ Bilirubin: ____

Most recent CBC: Goals→ Hgb/Hct: ____ Platelets: ____
Product replacement required? Bleeding? Local or Generalized

Lab Schedule: ACT q___h, Anti-Xa q___h, PTT q___h, PT/INR/Fibrinogen q___h, AT3 q___h, CBC q___h,
LD q___h, Plasma Free Hgb q___h, TEG q___h, Other ____

Current Gtts: ____

Fluid Balance: (if on CRRT, skip this)
0700 fluid balance: ____
Urine Output:____ml/kg/hr over last 24h

CRRT:
CRRT Day #: ____
Indication: ____
Vascath: ____ Filter: ____ Mode: ____
Settings:
BFR: ____
Dialysate Rate: ____
Replacement Rate: ____
Pre or Post: ____
Ordered Hourly Change: ____
Output as bonus? YES or NO
0700 Fluid Balance ____
Next scheduled filter change:____
Issues/Complications?
Urine Output: ____ml/kg/hr over last 24h
Lab Schedule: BMP/Mag/Phos q___h

Specialist to recap of plan/ECMO parameters reviewed, verify order updated if changes made:

- ECLS Daily Parameters (order to be updated if changes are made)
  Protocol: Hgb/Hct: CO2:
  Monitoring Lab: Platelets: Maps:
  Range for titration: paO2:
- ECLS flow, sweep, pump FiO2:
- Lab Schedule (order to be updated if change are made)
- Goal Fluid Balance for next 24 hours/Diuretics:
- Inotropic/vasopressors and other agent titration:
- Ventilatory Management/Are we ready for lung recruitment?
- Adjunct therapies: (CRRT/Apheresis)
- Procedures planned for the day?
- CXR/head US ordered for tomorrow?
- Recap any specialist concerns
- Other relevant goals?

Fig. 2. ECMO service line rounding tool. Nursing presentation rounding tool for the ECMO service line at Le Bonheur Children's Hospital in Memphis, Tennessee.

accurate and up-to-date information during multidisciplinary rounds, to ensure that orders and daily ECMO parameters were updated every 24 hours in the electronic medical record, to improve ECMO specialist engagement during rounds, and to provide a comprehensive overview of the ECMO patient's clinical status and plan of medical care. ECMO specialist-led rounds were met with enthusiasm and supported by the Critical Care division and implemented in ECMO patients within both the PICU and the CICU (**Fig. 3**).

Multidisciplinary Rounds in the Pediatric Intensive Care Unit

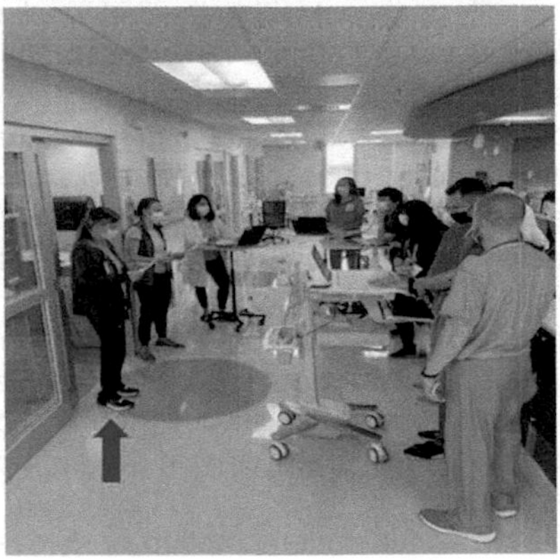

Fig. 3. Multidisciplinary rounds in the PICU. ECMO specialist (*arrow*) leading multidisciplinary rounds in the pediatric intensive unit at Le Bonheur children's Hospital in Memphis, Tennessee.

After the first 3 months of implementation, a survey using a 4-point Likert scale was disseminated to 32 ECMO specialists and 21 critical care attending physicians to evaluate ECMO specialist-led rounds. Response rates were at 62% for ECMO specialists and 66% for critical care attending physicians. Most notably, both groups reported 100% agreement in (1) improved communication between ECMO specialists and physicians, (2) improved ECMO specialist engagement in rounds, and (3) presentation of acute and up-to-date information. The rounding tool proved to be especially helpful when more than one medical team was involved in directing care of high-risk, dynamic patients, such as ECMO patients. Moreover, an additional benefit realized by the team is that the tool provides a structured format for ECMO specialist bedside hand-off. ECMO specialist-led rounds have been adopted by the institution and have been in successful implementation for more than 4 years.

Cardiac intensive care unit

The CICU at Le Bonheur Children's Hospital is a 10-bed unit dedicated to critically ill infants and children with congenital and acquired heart disease. Facilitators for the adoption of nurse-led rounds included a very strong culture valuing the nurse's role as part of the CICU team and well-established, consistent, and active nursing engagement during multidisciplinary rounds. Senior nurses and the medical team recognized that nurses in their first 2 years of practice needed more support in understanding their patient's unique cardiac physiology beyond cardiac illustrations displayed at the bedside. Thus, increasing novice nurse knowledge and critical thinking skills related to their patient's cardiac physiology was the motivating factor for implementing nurse-led rounds.

The medical provider team initiated the conversation of nurse-led rounds by approaching the CICU nursing practice council. Their request was met with interest, and a work group consisting of a charge nurse, unit-based nurse manager, and cardiac critical care attending was gathered to create the new rounding structure and associated nurse presentation tool. A distinctive feature of nurse-led rounds in the CICU model includes the opportunity for the bedside nurse to express their overall assessment of the patient's clinical status and their specific concerns for the day. By identifying nursing concerns on the front end of rounds, rather than the back end as is commonly done, the concerns are addressed during formulation of the medical plan in a more collaborative fashion.

Two challenges were readily apparent within the first week of implementation. First, much like the IMCU nurses, the CICU nurses were not amenable to the teaching style of the medical providers on rounds. They similarly felt that they were being belittled by being asked repetitive questions. Some nurses expressed that they felt embarrassed by not being able to easily answer questions meant to spark active discussion and learning. Others reported feeling judged for their lack of understanding of their patient's physiology and being exposed in a group setting. Teaching was adjusted by the providers to address the whole multidisciplinary team present during rounds. Small adjustments in the teaching medical provider's body positioning and eye contact were made to be directed at everyone rather than focused solely on the bedside nurse. These thoughtful maneuvers along with the modifications to the teaching style created an environment where the nurses were more comfortable and more apt to participate in the discussion.

The second barrier to successful implementation of nurse-led rounds was a small cohort of nurses who were resistant to practice change. A few seasoned critical care nurses viewed the practice change as unnecessary and would intentionally be unavailable to present or would be completely absent from the bedside. Also, a small cadre of novice nurses were overwhelmed by adding another layer of responsibility to their already busy and challenging daily practice. Change can cause fear and anxiety, and resistance to change is normal and should be expected. Clear and frequent communication from nursing leadership and the work group, along with opportunities for the nursing staff to provide feedback, mitigated the effects of those resistant to change and ensured that the new culture was sustainable. Last, real-time support during rounds through patience and coaching had the largest impact on improving nurse participation and buy-in.

Nurse-led rounds were implemented in 2019 and remain a mainstay of CICU nursing practice. Interestingly, the nursing presentation continues as originally developed yet the rounding tool is no longer in use. The practice has become so engrained in the culture that new nurses are trained on how to present the rounding information by using their own assessment and knowledge of the patient and the unit-based nursing hand-off sheet. Since the implementation of nurse-led rounds, the medical provider team has noticed a considerable increase in the bedside nurses' comprehension of the complex anatomy and physiology of congenital heart disease and their ability to apply that knowledge while caring for their patients.

Children's Hospital of Orange County Experience

The Children's Hospital of Orange County in Orange County, California is a 334-bed pediatric hospital affiliated with the University of California, Irvine. In 2018, their 18-bed PICU and 12-bed CICU implemented a nurse-led rounding tool to improve nursing presence during daily rounds. Nursing presence was often requested but not required at the time. A new structure for daily rounds, including the rounding tool (**Fig. 4**), was internally developed by a team consisting of dayshift critical care nurses, respiratory therapists, nurse practitioners, and critical care physicians. A pre-survey was conducted between June and July 2018 among the 2 critical care units,

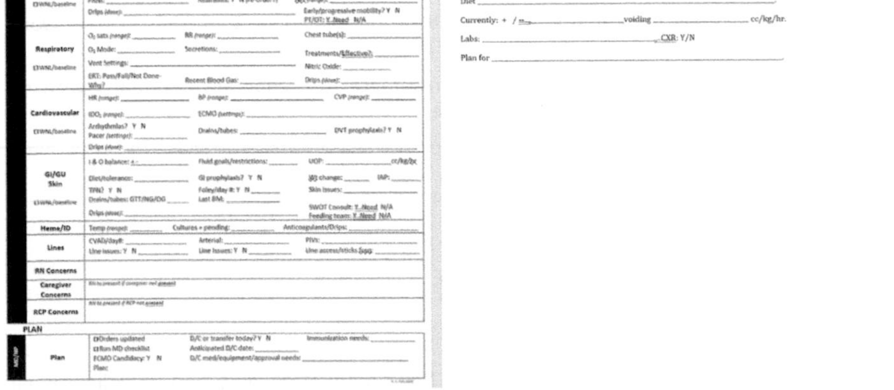

Pediatric Intensive Care Unit and Cardiac Intensive Care Unit Rounding Tool

CHOC Children's
PICU/CVICU Daily Rounding Tool
DATE: / /
Patient label

SUMMARY
H&P/Diagnosis/ ICU Course

ASSESSMENT
Labs/Tests: Critical/significant values only: ___ Last CXR: ___ Lab frequency: ___ Blood products past 24-hrs? Y N Scans in last 24-hrs? Y N
Neurological: Pain (range): ___ WAT-1: ___ Drains/monitors: ___ CAP-D: ___ ICP (range): ___ PRNs: ___ Restraints: Y N (re-order?) Drips (dose): ___ Early/progressive mobility? Y N PT/OT: Y Need N/A
Respiratory: O₂ sats (range): ___ RR (range): ___ Chest tube(s): ___ O₂ Mode: ___ Secretions: ___ Treatments/Effective?: ___ Vent Settings: ___ Nitric Oxide: ___ ERT: Pass/Fail/Not Done-Why? Recent Blood Gas: ___ Drips (dose): ___
Cardiovascular: HR (range): ___ BP (range): ___ CVP (range): ___ ECMO (settings): ___ Arrhythmias? Y N Pacer (settings): ___ Drains/tubes: ___ DVT prophylaxis? Y N Drips (dose): ___
GI/GU Skin: I & O balance: ___ Fluid goals/restrictions: ___ UOP: ___ cc/kg/hr Diet/tolerance: ___ GI prophylaxis? Y N IAP: ___ TPN? Y N Foley/day #: Y N ___ Skin issues: ___ Drains/tubes: GTT/NG/OG ___ Last BM: ___ SWOT Consult: Y Need N/A Drips (dose): ___ Feeding team: Y Need N/A
Heme/ID: Temp (range): ___ Cultures + pending: ___ Anticoagulants/Drips: ___
Lines: CVAD/day#: ___ Arterial: ___ PIVs: ___ Line issues: Y N ___ Line issues: Y N ___
RN Concerns
Caregiver Concerns
RCP Concerns

PLAN
Plan: Orders updated; Run MD checklist; ECMO Candidacy: Y N; Plan: D/C or transfer today? Y N; Anticipated D/C date: ___; D/C med/equipment/approval needs: ___; Immunization needs: ___

Cardiac Rounds:

Cardiac rounds are Monday through Friday. The team will go from 601-612 and it is the expectation that every RN is standing at their patient's door at 0645.

(Name) ___, ___ yrs/months old with (cardiac diagnosis) ___, now post op day ___ from (surgery) ___.

Or, admitted on (date) ___ for (admission): ___.

Overnight, vitals stable OR specific ranges if out of range: HR ___ BP ___/___

RR ___. On (room air or O2 device) ___ with sats ___%.

Diet ___.

Currently: + / ___ voiding ___ cc/kg/hr.

Labs: ___ CXR: Y/N

Plan for ___

Fig. 4. PICU and CICU rounding tool. Nursing presentation rounding tool for the pediatric and CICU at Children's Hospital Orange Country in Orange, California.

and its results were used to develop the new rounding structure. Nurse-led rounding structure included a brief patient history, acute events from the previous 24 hours, pertinent laboratory data, and physical assessment by systems.

Staff education on the new rounding structure, delivered by the PICU and CICU nursing practice councils, occurred for approximately 3 months. The nurse-led rounding structure with the new rounding tool was piloted in the CICU in December 2018 and disseminated to the PICU in May 2019. Post-implementation surveys were conducted at 6 and 12 months. Most of those surveyed responded and reported a positive overall experience with nurse-led multidisciplinary rounds. Survey results were most remarkable for noting nurse availability to present during rounds, the positive impact of nurse presence throughout the entirety of rounds, nurse ability to anticipate when rounds for their patient would commence, and the overall length of rounds. Nurse-led rounds in the PICU at Children's Hospital of Orange County generated a new culture that places prominent value on the bedside nurse's role in the multidisciplinary team.

SUMMARY

PICUs are complex settings that demand high-level team dynamics for optimal patient outcomes. The paradigm shift from provider to nurse-led multidisciplinary rounds can enhance collaboration in patient care, but teams who adopt this model must anticipate barriers to implementation. The 4 service lines outlined above navigated resistance to change from both global and individual perspectives. In doing so, they promoted cultures of mutual value and respect that are a substrate for cohesive, efficient patient care. Nurse-led rounds further validate the bedside nurse as the patient expert and promote a sense of autonomy in nursing practice, essential factors to satisfaction and longevity in a nursing career. Opportunity for future work lies in exploring the longitudinal outcomes of nurse-led rounds' effects on patients and teams.

CLINICS CARE POINTS

- Nurse-led rounds are an effective model for increasing nurse engagement and collaboration in a high-risk, multidisciplinary environment.
- Nurse presentation of patients during rounds should be unit-tailored and guided by a formal presentation tool.
- An effective formal presentation tool should be developed by a multidisciplinary work group.
- Anticipating and planning for barriers and resistance to change are essential aspects of implementing positive clinical practice change.

DISCLOSURES

The authors have no disclosures to declare.

REFERENCES

1. Baggs JG, Ryan SA, Phelps CE, et al. The association between interdisciplinary collaboration and patient outcomes in a medical intensive care unit. Heart Lung 1992;21:18–24.

2. Institute of Medicine (US). Committee on quality of Health care in America. In: Kohn LT, Corrigan JM, Donaldson MS, editors. To err is human: building a safer health system. Washington (DC): National Academies Press (US); 2000.
3. Donchin Y, Gopher D, Olin M, et al. A look into the nature and causes of human errors in the intensive care unit. Crit Care Med 1995;23(2):294–300.
4. Dittman K, Hughes S. Increased nursing participation in multidisciplinary rounds to enhance communication, patient safety, and parent satisfaction. Crit Care Nurs Clin North Am 2018;30(4):445–55.e4.
5. Acal Jiménez R, Swartz M, McCorkle R. Improving quality through nursing participation at bedside rounds in a pediatric acute care unit: a pilot project. J Pediatr Nurs 2018;43:45–55.
6. Reeves S, Pelone F, Harrison R, et al. Interprofessional collaboration to improve professional practice and healthcare outcomes. Cochrane Database Syst Rev 2017;6(6):CD000072.
7. The Joint Commission. 2017 National Patient Safety Goals. Available at: https://www.jointcommission.org/assets/1/6/2017_NPSG_HAP_ER.pdf. Accessed May 1, 2023.
8. Gonzalo JD, Kuperman E, Lehman E, et al. Bedside interprofessional rounds: perceptions of benefits and barriers by internal medicine nursing staff, attending physicians, and housestaff physicians. J Hosp Med 2014;9(10):646–51.
9. Burns K. Nurse-physician rounds: a collaborative approach to improving communication, efficiencies, and perception of care. Medsurg Nurs 2011;20(4):194–9.
10. Katkin JP, Kressly SJ, Edwards AR, et al. Guiding principles for team-based pediatric care. Pediatrics 2017;140(2):e20171489.
11. Rosen P, Stenger E, Bochkoris M, et al. Family-centered multidisciplinary rounds enhance the team approach in pediatrics. Pediatrics 2009;123(4):e603–8.
12. Subramony A, Hametz PA, Balmer D. Family-centered rounds in theory and practice: an ethnographic case study. Acad Pediatr 2014;14(2):200–6.
13. Chew BH, Tang CJ, Lim WS, et al. Interprofessional bedside rounds: nurse-physician collaboration and perceived barriers in an Asian hospital. J Interprof Care 2019;33(6):820–2.
14. Mullen J, Reynolds M, Marante A, et al. Nurse-integrated rounds improve communication in the pediatric intensive care unit. Crit Care Med 2019;47(1):688.
15. Sharma A, Norton L, Gage S, et al. A quality improvement initiative to achieve high nursing presence during patient- and family-centered rounds. Hosp Pediatr 2014;4(1):1–5.
16. Tang CJ, Zhou WT, Chan SW, et al. Interprofessional collaboration between junior doctors and nurses in the general ward setting: a qualitative exploratory study. J Nurs Manag 2018;26(1):11–8.
17. Aitken LM, Burmeister E, Clayton S, et al. The impact of Nursing Rounds on the practice environment and nurse satisfaction in intensive care: pre-test post-test comparative study. Int J Nurs Stud 2011;48(8):918–25.
18. Gormley DK, Costanzo AJ, Goetz J, et al. Impact of nurse-led interprofessional rounding on patient experience. Nurs Clin North Am 2019;54(1):115–26.
19. Dietz AS, Pronovost PJ, Mendez-Tellez PA, et al. A systematic review of teamwork in the intensive care unit: what do we know about teamwork, team tasks, and improvement strategies? J Crit Care 2014;29(6):908–14.
20. Pritts KE, Hiller LG. Implementation of physician and nurse patient rounding on a 42-bed medical unit. Medsurg Nurs 2014;23(6):408–13.
21. Adams HA, Feudale RM. Implementation of a structured rounding tool for interprofessional care team rounds to improve communication and collaboration in patient

care. Pediatr Nurs 2018;44(5):229–46. Available at: https://search-ebscohost-com.ezproxy.uthsc.edu/login.aspx?direct=true&db=ccm&AN=132450461&site=ehost-live. Accessed May 18, 2023.

22. Bartram T, Joiner TA, Stanton P. Factors affecting the job stress and job satisfaction of Australian nurses: implications for recruitment and retention. Contemp Nurse 2004;17(3):293–304.

23. Gausvik C, Lautar A, Miller L, et al. Structured nursing communication on interdisciplinary acute care teams improves perceptions of safety, efficiency, understanding of care plan and teamwork as well as job satisfaction. J Multidiscip Healthc 2015;8:33–7. Published 2015 Jan 14,

Asthma Care Protocol Implementation in the Pediatric Intensive Care Unit

Exie Meredith, DNP, APRN, CPNP-AC[a],*,
Jenilea Thomas, APRN, MSN, CPNP AC/PC, NNP[b]

KEYWORDS

- Pediatric • Asthma management • Asthma • Pediatric intensive care

KEY POINTS

- Asthma affects nearly 7 million children in the United States.
- Asthma is an inflammatory disorder that causes airway obstruction, bronchospasms, and mucus plugging.
- Asthma exacerbations are episodes of progressive shortness of breath, coughing, wheezing, and chest tightness.
- Treatment in the pediatric intensive care unit includes administration of bronchodilators, magnesium sulfate, and steroids. Other therapies include the use of noninvasive positive pressure, endotracheal intubation, mechanical ventilation, and in severe cases the use of anesthesia gasses and extracorporeal membrane oxygenation.

INTRODUCTION

Asthma is a complex disease characterized as an inflammatory disorder causing airflow obstruction due to inflammation, bronchospasms, and mucus plugging.[1] Identification and proper management of asthma is crucial to prevent longer term outcomes. Asthma affects approximately 7 million children and is frequently the reason for hospital admissions and pediatric intensive care unit (PICU) stays.[2] Asthma can be managed outpatient for the majority of patients but for those with severe asthma and recurrent exacerbations, it can be life-threatening. Asthma exacerbations present usually with increasing shortness of breath, wheezing, chest tightness, and cough. Status asthmaticus is a condition where patients do not respond to first-tier therapies and are at risk of progressing to respiratory failure. Patients who present with status asthmaticus have failed to respond to first-line rescue therapies and require continued treatments or advanced therapies usually require admission to the PICU. A history of

[a] Baylor College of Medicine, 1 Baylor Plaza, Houston, TX, USA; [b] Texas Children's Hospital, 6651 Main Street, MC E1420, Houston, TX 77030, USA
* Corresponding author. 6651 Main Street, MC E1420, Houston, TX, 77030.
E-mail address: exmeredi@texaschildrens.org

Crit Care Nurs Clin N Am 35 (2023) 337–346
https://doi.org/10.1016/j.cnc.2023.04.007
0899-5885/23/© 2023 Elsevier Inc. All rights reserved.

severe exacerbations and previous hospital and ICU admissions is a risk factor for subsequent ICU admission.[3] In 2020, two hundred pediatric deaths were attributed to asthma in the United States.[4]

HISTORY

Asthma is the most common chronic illness in children and affects approximately 8.5% of children in the United States.[5] There is an increased prevalence of asthma among black children, compared with white children, as well as those in lower socioeconomic statuses and urban environments.[6] Literature has shown that Black Americans are 3 times more likely to die from asthma.[4]

Many children can wheeze with viral respiratory infections but not all of them will have childhood asthma. Most infants who wheeze do not have an increased risk of asthma later in life. Long-term follow-up studies have shown that approximately 30% of cases where wheezing begins before the child is aged 1 year have significantly poorer pulmonary function tests than those who never experienced wheezing.[7] There are different phenotypes that have been identified to predict childhood asthma, from transient wheezing to persistent wheezing with peak flow variability and hyperresponsiveness. An asthma predictive index (API) was developed by Castro-Rodriguez to evaluate children with wheezing.[5] This tool was made to identify children at risk for asthma and identify subgroups with recurrent wheezing at greatest risk. This tool can be used while obtaining admission history on your patients to help evaluate their risks. It is recommended that this tool is used to decide whether to initiate controller therapy in children aged from 0 to 4 years.

Asthma Predictive Index

- Identify high-risk children (aged 2–3 years)[5]:
- Greater than or equal to wheezing episodes in the past year (at least one must be diagnosed by a provider)

PLUS

- One Major criterion:
  Parents with asthma
  Atopic dermatitis
  Aero-allergen sensitivity

OR

- Two minor criteria
  Food sensitivity
  Peripheral eosinophilia (>4%)
  Wheezing not related to infection

Genetic factors are important but it is thought to be unlikely that a single gene is responsible for asthma. Children with a strong family history are at an increased risk of developing asthma. Several possible genes have been proposed for genetic linkage but it has been found that asthma is both a genetical and phenotypical heterogeneous disorder.[2]

API, along with careful physical examination and history, as well as the patient's response to treatment, is required for diagnosis. Spirometry is recommended for diagnosis but not all children are able to complete this testing depending on developmental level and age. Environmental factors play a role as well. There are many theories to explain asthma prevalence. One theory suggests an apparent association between exposure to irritants, such as second-hand tobacco smoke, viruses, and pollen with the subsequent development of asthma.[2] There is also a related theory regarding early exposure to respiratory syncytial virus being linked to the development of asthma.[5] Other theories include the "hygiene hypothesis" and the immunologic paradigm.[2] The study of the origins and causes of asthma are still ongoing.

PATHOPHYSIOLOGY

Asthma is defined as chronic inflammation of the lower airways with bronchial hyperreactivity, smooth muscle contractions, and airway obstruction resulting in edema or mucus plugging.[1,8,9] There are various triggers that can cause asthma attacks such as allergens, exercise, respiratory infections, psychological stress, and inhaled irritants.[9] This leads to an inflammatory cell response and a subsequent mediator release that leads to bronchial inflammation and airway edema. The inflammation process causes wheezing, chest tightness, and coughing, which is due to air trapping or obstruction.[1] The air trapping leads to high lung volumes, decreased lung compliance, and hypoxemia. As lung compliance worsens, negative pressure creates pulmonary edema. Hypoxemia also occurs and is related to the ventilation-perfusion mismatch. The continued hypoxemia results in anaerobic cellular metabolism, which is shown as metabolic acidosis.[8] If treatment is not initiated, the increased work of breathing, respiratory muscle fatigue, and hypoxia will lead to respiratory failure.[9]

DEFINITION/DIAGNOSTIC CRITERIA (DEGREE OF SEVERITY)

Table 1.

PHYSICAL EXAMINATION/DIAGNOSTIC EVALUATION

Physical Examination:
- Vital signs: pulse, heart rate, oxygen saturation, respiratory rate
  - Tachycardia usually seen, especially if already received bronchodilators
- Responsiveness/alertness
- Ability to complete a sentence
  - Mild: Speaks in complete sentence
  - Moderate: Speaks in short or partial sentences
  - Severe: Speaks in short phrases or single words
- Exhaustion level
- Color: pink, pale, cyanotic
- Lung sounds: wheezing, chest expansion equally, and adequate breath sounds bilaterally
  - Widespread audible expiratory wheezing
  - Worsening symptoms are decreased breath sounds, no air movement, or silent chest
- Dyspnea
  - Frequently cannot complete a sentence in one breath or is too breathless to feed/talk
- Use of accessory muscles
  - Mild: No retractions to mild intercostal retractions
  - Moderate: Moderate intercostal or substernal retractions
  - Severe: Moderate intercostal or substernal retractions with nasal flaring
- Rhinitis, nasal polyps, mucosal swelling

Table 1
GINA (Global Initiative for Asthma)-diagnostic criteria for asthma in adults, adolescents, and children aged 6 to 11 y

1 History of variable respiratory symptoms

Feature	Symptoms or features that support the diagnosis of asthma
Wheeze, shortness of breath, chest tightness and cough (Descriptors may vary between cultures and by age)	• More than one type of respiratory symptom (in adults, isolated cough is seldom due to asthma) • Symptoms occur variably over time and vary in intensity • Symptoms are often worse at night or on waking • Symptoms are often triggered by exercise, laughter, allergens, cold air Symptoms often appear or worsen with viral infections

2 Confirmed variable expiratory airflow limitation

Feature	Consideration, definitions, criteria
2.1 Documented [a] expiratory airflow limitation	At a time when FEV_1 (forced exhalation volume in one second) is reduced, confirm that FEV_1/FVC (forced vital capacity) is reduced compared with the lower limit of normal (it is usually >0.75–0.80 in adults, >0.90 in children[17])
AND	
2.2 Documented [a] excessive variability in lung function[a](one or more of the following):	The greater the variations or the more occasions excess variation is seen, the more confident the diagnosis. If initially negative, tests can be repeated during symptoms or in the early morning
• Positive bronchodilator (BD) responsiveness (reversibility) test	The greater the variations, or the more occasions excess variation is seen, the more confident the diagnosis. If initially negative, tests can be repeated during symptoms or in the early morning
• Excessive variability in twice-daily PEF during 2 wk	*Adults:* increase in FEV_1 of >12% and >200 mL (greater confidence if increase is >15% and >400 mL). *Children:* increase in FEV_1 of >12% predicted Measure change 10–15 min after 200–400 mcg salbutamol (albuterol) or equivalent, compared with pre-BD readings. Positive test more likely if BD withheld before test: SABA $\geq$4 h, twice-daily LABA 24 h, once-daily LABA 36 h
• Significant increase in lung function after 4 wk of anti-inflammatory treatment	Adults: average daily diurnal PEF variability >10%[a] Children: average daily diurnal PEF variability >13%[a]
• Positive exercise challenge test	*Adults:* increase in FEV_1 by >12% and > 200 mL (or PEF[b] by > 20%) from baseline after 4 wk of treatment, outside respiratory infections
• Positive bronchial challenge test (usually only for adults)	Fall in FEV_1 from baseline of $\geq$12% with standard soese of methacholine, or $\geq$ 15% with standardized hyperventilation, hypertonic saline or mannitol challenge

(continued on next page)

Table 1
(continued)
• Excessive variation in lung function between visits (good specificity but poor sensitivity) — *Adults:* variation in FEV_1 of >12% and >200 mL between visits, outside of respiratory infections *Children:* variation in FEV_1 of >12% in FEV_1 or > 15% in PEF^b between visits (may include respiratory infections)

See Box 1 to 3(p.26) for how to confirm the diagnosis in patients already taking controller treatment.

Abbreviations: BD, Bronchodilator (SABA or rapid-acting LABA); FEV_1, forced expiratory volume in 1 s; ICS, inhaled corticosteroid; LABA, long-acting beta$_2$-agonist; PEF, peak expiratory flow (highest of 3 readings); SABA, short-acting beta$_2$-agonist.

[a] Daily diurnal PEF variability is calculated from twice daily PEF as (day's highest minus day's lowest) divided by (mean of day's highest and lowest), averaged during 1 week.

[b] For PEF, use the same meter each time, as PEF may vary by up to 20% between different meters. BD responsiveness may be lost during severe exacerbations or viral infections and airflow limitation may become persistent over time. If reversibility is not present at initial presentation, the next step depends on the availability of other tests and the urgency of the need for treatment. In a situation of clinical urgency, asthma treatment may be commenced and diagnostic testing arranged within the next few weeks (Box 1–4, p.27) but other conditions that can mimic asthma (Box-5) should be considered, and the diagnosis confirmed as soon as possible.

Data Source: [Global Initiative for Asthma. Global Strategies for Asthma Management and Prevention. 2022. Available at: https://ginasthma.org/wp-content/uploads/2022/07/GINA-Main-Report-2022-FINAL-22-07-01-WMS.pdf. Accessed December 31st, 2022.]

Diagnosis:
- History:
  - Severity and duration of symptoms
  - Medications
  - Level of asthma control
  - Family history of asthma
  - Triggers
    - Cigarette smoke
    - Allergens
    - Environmental triggers
    - Exercise
    - Respiratory infections
    - Psychological stress
    - Inhaled irritants
- Imaging
  - CXR
    - Usually shows hyperinflation due to air trapping
- Laboratory test
  - Blood gas
    - Early stage: mild hypocapnia
    - Worsens as the patient fatigues and develop impending respiratory failure
  - Viral panel (based on symptoms)
- Testing (usually done outpatient)
  - Lung function test
  - Allergy testing

WHAT QUALIFIES A PEDIATRIC INTENSIVE CARE UNIT ADMISSION?

Acute asthma exacerbations vary in severity and response to treatment. Patients that are not responsive to first-line treatments and needing additional treatments, including but not limited to noninvasive positive pressure, intravenous terbutaline, continuous albuterol with increasing work of breathing, and of course, mechanical ventilation, require PICU admission. Severe asthma, prior hospital, and PICU admissions are risk factors for subsequent PICU admissions. One study on PICU admissions found that most patients with near-fatal exacerbations have severe asthma, and having multiple admissions is a risk factor for PICU admissions. More asthmatics that are admitted to the ICU have severe persistent asthma.[10]

GUIDELINES

The National Asthma Education and Prevention Program guidelines recommend treating 3 main goals.[10]

1. Correcting hypoxia
2. Reversal of airflow obstruction
3. Reduction of relapse and future.

They have categorized treatment therapies into first, second, and third lines.

First-tier treatment therapies include oxygen, fluids, inhaled beta-agonist, inhaled anticholinergics, and intravenous corticosteroids.

Patients with acute exacerbations have ventilation-perfusion (VQ) mismatch, which results in hypoxia commonly, which is frequently corrected with minimal oxygen. Oxygen is a first-line therapy in acute exacerbations.[10]

Intravenous (IV) fluids are an important treatment in status asthmaticus. Children with asthma have hypovolemia due to insensible losses. These insensible losses can come from tachypnea, increased metabolic activity due to increased work of breathing and those patients that may have viral or bacterial triggers and fevers. Euvolemia is the goal of fluid replacement.[10]

Short-acting inhaled beta-agonists (SABA) are one of the primary treatment therapies for acute asthma exacerbations. Albuterol is the most commonly used beta agonist. Aerosol delivery of albuterol depends on dose, gas flow, and device used to deliver the medication plus the child's respiratory effort; due to this, metered dose inhalers are the preferred method of delivery over nebulization.[2] However, when patients are not responding to albuterol every 2 hours and need more frequent administration, continuous albuterol via nebulization is the next step. Albuterol commonly has side effects that should be monitored including tachycardia, restlessness, anxiety, stomachache, tremors, and hypokalemia.[11] Hypokalemia is a side effect of high dose or prolonged use of albuterol. It results from intracellular potassium shifts due to skeletal muscle beta receptor activation, although it does normalize quickly after discontinuing albuterol. It is a concern for patients with high doses or frequent doses of beta agonists, such as albuterol.[10] Therefore, it is crucial to follow serum chemistry levels in these patients.

Ipratropium is an inhaled anticholinergic drug used as an adjunct treatment of acute asthma exacerbations. It blocks cholinergic receptors, decreases cholinergic bronchomotor tone, and decreases mucosal edema and secretions.[10] Ipratropium is given in conjunction with a SABA, usually albuterol, and is shown to be most effective in the emergency department (ED) setting. Use after the ED in the inpatient setting has not been shown to have more benefits.

Systemic corticosteroids are another primary treatment of acute asthma exacerbations. The use of corticosteroids decreases inflammation and mucus production, and it is shown to enhance the efficacy of bronchodilators.[10] Patients with severe asthma should receive their first dose of steroids on presentation.[2] In the ED setting, oral dosing is acceptable, with recommendations for prednisolone or prednisone orally for 1 to 2 doses. Patients requiring PICU admission will receive intravenous administration; methylprednisolone is the most common corticosteroid used.[2] Steroids are prescribed cautiously due to side effects but they are necessary for a short course in severe asthma. If used for a short course, they do not need to be tapered or weaned before stopping. Common side effects of IV steroids to be aware of when caring for patients with asthma include increased appetite, upset stomach, insomnia, and confusion.[12]

Second-tier therapies: IV magnesium, Heliox, IV beta agonist, high-flow nasal cannula (HFNC), noninvasive ventilation (NIV).

IV magnesium sulfate ($MgSO_4$) is another adjunctive therapy considered when patients are not responsive to first-line treatments. Magnesium sulfate acts as a smooth muscle relaxer and relieves bronchoconstriction.[10] It also works by reducing histamine and prostaglandin release.[2] The recommended dose is 25 to 50 mg/kg for the treatment of severe asthma. Hypotension is a potential side effect of magnesium administration due to the smooth muscle relaxation of the vascular bed. This side effect is uncommon but can be easily treated with fluid boluses.

Heliox is an inert gas that produces favorable gas flow. Heliox leads to less turbulence through narrow airways and can be used to deliver nebulized beta-agonists. Studies have shown heliox does not benefit patients with mild or moderate exacerbations but in severe and very severe exacerbations, there were improvements in hospitalizations and severity scores.[10]

IV beta-agonist can be used as well. Theoretically, they may be superior in drug delivery when bronchial constriction is so severe that it may prevent aerosolized drugs from reaching the distal airways.[2] IV terbutaline is the most commonly used IV beta agonist. This medication can be titrated to effect, although it is more likely to have beta-agonist side effects.[2]

HFNC can be used when patients require more respiratory support than is given with a simple nasal cannula or facemask. HFNC provides heated, humidified, high-flow oxygen therapy via a nasal cannula and can deliver up to 60 L/min of flow.[13] HFNC delivers a flow at a rate that is higher than inspiratory demands, which provides minimal end distending pressures and increased residual functional capacity.[13] HFNC has also been shown to generate nasopharyngeal pressure, reduce airway resistance, and flush dead space in the nasopharyngeal area, enhancing carbon dioxide clearance.[13] High-flow nasal cannula can be used in combination with aerosolized continuous albuterol. In a new study (2021), HFNC performed similarly to a face mask for the delivery of albuterol.[14] There are no clear guidelines for set flow rate in pediatrics; flows of 1 to 2 L/kg/min are used for patients up to 10 kg, then 0.5 L/kg/min above 10 kg.[13]

Bi-level airway positive pressure (BiPAP) or other noninvasive ventilation is recommended for patients with acute exacerbations who have not improved with the previously mentioned therapies. Positive pressure ventilation opens distal airways and exposes more B-adrenergic receptors, and it offloads increased work of breathing caused by autopeeping. NIV can reduce respiratory work, improve atelectasis, and promote collateral ventilation.[2] Although it can increase air-trapping and VQ mismatching.[10] BiPAP works well for those with severe exacerbations who are fatigued or approaching respiratory failure. It is used in an effort to avoid intubation.

Third-tier therapies: IV ketamine, mechanical ventilation/intubation, inhaled anesthetics, ECMO.

IV Ketamine is a sedation that is used frequently during the intubation of asthmatic patients. It can be used in the preintubation period as a sedative, and it produces bronchodilation. There are studies to use ketamine for severe exacerbations looking at its role in avoiding respiratory failure/intubation.[10]

Patients with status asthmaticus have increased airway resistance. This resistance to airflow increases work of breathing that leads to increased stress and effort.[10] Gas trapping increases, which is also known as dynamic hyperinflation, and limits full exhalation. In status asthmaticus, exhalation is decreased by airway resistance, and the time to exhale is lengthened. This results in air trapping in the alveoli at the end of exhalation/before inhalation.

Endotracheal intubation is used for those patients with hypoxia, hypercarbia, altered mental status, and exhaustion. Clinical judgment is used to determine the correct time for intubation for those patients with hypercarbia, altered mental status, and perceived tiredness alone is nonspecific and should be deterd on an indi. Usually, severe hypercarbia, apnea, and coma are definitive indications for intubation. Complications can develop in mechanical ventilation with the asthmatic. As the gas is trapped in the alveoli at the end of expiration, the alveolar pressure increases, which can lead to baro-volutrauma and pneumothoraces, as well as pneumomediastinum.[10] When intrathoracic pressure increases, right atrial pressure decreases and venous return decreases.

Inhaled anesthetics can be used as a rescue therapy for patients with severe life-threatening asthma exacerbations. Inhaled agents, such as isoflurane, have bronchodilatory effects, decrease airway responsiveness, and decrease histamine-induced bronchospasms.[15] These medications have risks and the PICUs that utilize them should have specific protocols for their usage involving collaboration with respiratory therapy and anesthesia. Inhaled anesthetics require endotracheal intubation, the proper equipment, and trained staff. The main side effect of using anesthesia gasses is hypotension and many patients using inhaled gasses for asthma treatment will require administration of IV vasopressors.[15]

Extracorporeal membrane oxygenation (ECMO) allows the lungs to rest, and it is used in situations of near fatal asthma with persistent hypercapnic respiratory acidosis.[4] Placing the asthmatic patient on ECMO allows for bronchiolar relaxation. This is generally used after all previously mentioned therapies have been trialed. ECMO is an important option for refractory respiratory failure. A recent study of children with near fatal asthma showed a high survival rate for those that used inhaled anesthetics and/or ECMO. Patients supported with ECMO had less cumulative bronchodilator use.[4]

USE OF SCORE BASED RESPIRATORY DRIVEN PATHWAYS AND PROTOCOLS FOR ASTHMA CARE

Management of acute asthma is a multidisciplinary task. Many facilities have pathways and protocols to standardize care, enhance quality, and reduce unnecessary therapies. These pathways and protocols have been shown to decrease the length of stay and shorten the duration of continuous albuterol use.[16] These protocols can be used so that respiratory therapists and nursing can drive the weaning of albuterol treatments. Different respiratory scoring tools have been validated and are reliable, and these will vary between institutions. The ability to wean albuterol without the delay of waiting for a provider to assess the patient in a busy unit is a considerable advantage to having a weaning protocol.[17]

SUMMARY

Asthma is a complex chronic disease characterized by inflammatory disorder causing airflow obstruction due to inflammation, bronchospasms, and mucus plugging. Proper identification and management are crucial in preventing the development of irreversible airway changes and reducing morbidity and mortality in young children. Children who fail to respond to initial first-line therapies often require hospitalization, and many with severe exacerbations and near fatal asthma require admission to the PICU. Nursing care of these patients in the PICU requires close monitoring and excellent assessment of their respiratory status. Treatment of asthmatic patients in the PICU can range from continuous albuterol and steroid therapies to more advanced treatments such as BiPAP, mechanical ventilation, use of volatile gasses and even ECMO.

CLINICS CARE POINTS

- Asthma is a complex chronic disease of the lower airways.
- Wheezing episodes in children should initially be managed by an inhaled short-acting beta-agonist.
- Not all children who wheeze early in life with a respiratory illness will develop asthma.
- API is used along with history and physical examinations to diagnose asthma.
- There is increased prevalence of asthma in Black children.
- PICU admissions for status asthmaticus occur due to the need for second-line therapies, BiPAP, intubation, mechanical ventilation, shock, or respiratory failure, this will vary between hospitals and PICUs.
- Close assessment of respiratory status is important
  - Careful auscultation of breath sounds
  - Alert providers if decreased breath sounds, or silent chest
  - A silent chest with minimal airflow is a critical finding.
- Steroids should be administered on presentation to the hospital.
- Atrovent and ipratropium should be given alongside SABAs and is not proven to be effective outside of the emergency center (EC) setting.
- Respiratory driven albuterol weaning protocols have been proven safe and decrease the length of stay for patients with asthma.

DISCLOSURE

The authors have no financial relationships or conflict of interest relevant to this article to disclose.

REFERENCES

1. Global Initiative for Asthma. Global Strategies for Asthma Management and Prevention. 2022. Available at : https://ginasthma.org/wp-content/uploads/2022/07/GINA-Main-Report-2022-FINAL-22-07-01-WMS.pdf. Accessed December 31st, 2022.
2. Wong R, Maffei FA. Severe asthma. In: Lucking SE, Maffei FA, Tamburro RF, et al, editors. Pediatric critical care. Cham, Switzerland: Springer; 2021. p. 219–49.
3. Elizur A, Bacharier L, Strunk R. Pediatric asthma admissions: chronic severity and acute exacerbations. J Asthma 2007;44:285–9.
4. Custer C, O'Neil E, Paskaradevan J, et al. Children with near-fatal asthma: the use of inhaled volatile anesthetics and extracorporeal membrane oxygenation. Pediatric allergy, immunology, and pulmonology 2022;25(4):170–3.

5. Herzog R, Cunningham-Rundles S. Pediatric asthma: natural history, assessment and treatment. MSJM (Mt Sinai J Med) 2001;646–60. https://doi.org/10.1002/MSJ.

6. Kane N. Revealing the racial and spatial disparity in pediatric asthma: a Kansas City case study. Soc Sci Med 2020;292:114543.

7. Vega-Briceño L.E., Contreras Estay I. and Sánchez I., Children with recurrent wheezing, In: Bertrand P. and Sánchez I., *Pediatric respiratory diseases*, 2020, Springer; Cham, Switzerland, 205-214.

8. Hiday R, Abbott K. Pulmonary care: asthma guideline updates. Lenexa (KS): ACCP; 2022. p. 7–36. ACSAP 2022 Book 1).

9. Pediatric fundamental critical care support. 2nd edition. Society of Critical Care Medicine; 2011. p. 0–5.

10. Jones B, Fleming G, Otillio J, et al. Pediatric acute asthma exacerbations: evaluation and management from emergency department to intensive care unit. J Asthma 2016;53(6):607–17. https://doi.org/10.3109/02770903.2015.1067323.

11. Johnson DB, Merrell BJ, Bounds CG. Albuterol. [Updated 2022 sep 24]. In: stat pearls [internet]. Treasure Island (FL): Stat Pearls Publishing; 2022. Available at: https://www.ncbi.nlm.nih.gov/books/NBK482272/.

12. Grennan D, Wang S. Steroid side effects. JAMA 2019;322(3):282. https://doi.org/10.1001/jama.2019.8506.

13. Chao K, Chien Y, Mu S. High-flow nasal cannula in children with asthma exacerbation: a review of current evidence. Paediatr Respir Rev 2021;40:52–7.

14. Gates R, Haynes K, Rehder K, et al. High-flow nasal cannula in pediatric critical asthma. Respir Care 2021;66(8):1240–6.

15. Wong J, Lee J, Turner D, et al. A review of the use of adjunctive therapies in severe acute asthma exacerbation in critically ill children. Expet Rev Respir Med 2014;8(4):423–41. https://doi.org/10.1586/17476348.2014.915752.

16. Willis L, Danner N, Lloyd T, et al. Safe and effective use of score-based continuous albuterol therapy in a pathway for treatment of pediatric asthma. Respir Care 2022;67(11):1396–404.

17. Maue D, Tori A, Beardsley A, et al. Implementing a respiratory therapist-drive Continuous albuterol weaning protocol in the pediatric ICU. Respir Care 2019; 64(11):1358–65.

Battling Alarm Fatigue in the Pediatric Intensive Care Unit

Heather Herrera, RN, MSN, CPNP-AC/PC[a],
Danielle Wood, DNP, CPNP-AC[b],*

KEYWORDS

- Alarm fatigue • PICU • Alarm parameters • Actionable alarms • Desensitization

KEY POINTS

- Pediatric intensive care unit (PICU) nurses can be exposed to hundreds of alarms per shift, the majority of which are nonactionable.
- Alarm fatigue can cause desensitization to future alarms and negatively affect reaction time.
- Strategies should be used to decrease false and nonactionable alarms in the PICU.

HISTORY

The inception of critical care is tied to the origin of the nursing profession with Florence Nightingale requiring more severely ill soldiers in the Crimean War to be placed nearer to nurses' stations for closer monitoring.[1] It was not until the 1920s that Johns Hopkins Hospital in Baltimore, Maryland, opened a dedicated unit with 3 beds for neurosurgical patients requiring close postoperative observation.[1] With the devastating number of patients requiring artificial respiratory support during the polio epidemic in Copenhagen, Denmark, in the 1950s, it became evident that specialized care areas for patients requiring mechanical support were needed.[2] With the advent of specialized care areas, bedside cardiac telemetry monitoring was born within cardiac care units in the 1960s.[3,4] Pulse oximetry was developed in the 1970s but could not be translated to bedside monitoring until the 1980s, when smaller computer processors became available.[5] As technology continued to develop in the 1990s and 2000s, more and more sophisticated and invasive monitoring tools became available within intensive care units, including but not limited to invasive blood pressure monitoring, end-tidal carbon dioxide, and near-infrared spectroscopy.[1,4]

Pediatric intensive care units (PICUs) are busy areas of patient care, notorious for ongoing noises at all times, day and night. The patients in the PICU are often critically

[a] Christus Children's, 333 North, Santa Rosa Street, San Antonio, TX 78207, USA; [b] Duke University Hospital, 104 Lanier Valley Drive, Durham, NC 27703, USA
* Corresponding author. 2301 Erwin Road, Durham, NC 27710, USA.
E-mail address: Danielle.wood@duke.edu

Crit Care Nurs Clin N Am 35 (2023) 347–355
https://doi.org/10.1016/j.cnc.2023.05.003
0899-5885/23/© 2023 Elsevier Inc. All rights reserved.
ccnursing.theclinics.com

ill and require continual vigilant monitoring. These patients are at risk for acute, life-threatening conditions that require intensive supportive therapies and treatment. This may include conditions such as trauma, acute disease, and organ failure. Endo-tracheal intubation, central venous line placement, inotropic medication infusion, and renal replacement therapies are just a few of the invasive treatments that may be needed for treating these children. The purpose of these therapies is to help the child's body function through a life-threatening illness or injury.[6] Monitors are used in these patients to alert providers of changes in patient status with audible alarms. These alarms notify health-care personnel that the patient may need immediate intervention. Alarm fatigue occurs when health-care providers are exposed to so many alarms that they become desensitized to them. This desensitization leads to alarm apathy, delaying response time to critical changes in patient condition, which can negatively affect patients and their safety.[7] According to UR Health laboratory, studies have also demonstrated that with task interruption, such as a nurse responding to an alarm in the middle of drawing up a medication, the likelihood of a mistake occurring after the resumption of the initial activity is 25%.[8] This shows that alarms and health-care provider fatigue from those alarms are not the only threat that alarms pose to patient safety.

Current monitoring in the PICU includes, at minimum, heart rate, respiratory rate, blood pressure, temperature, and pulse oximetry. Other potential modalities of monitoring include intracranial pressure, central venous pressure, invasive arterial blood pressure, abdominal pressure, core body temperature, and cerebral and renal Somanetics. These monitors are meant to be sensitive to minute changes in patient condition, alerting staff and promoting quick intervention to these changes. Although alerting personnel to changes in condition can be beneficial, monitors lack the intuitive sensitivity to appropriately recognize individual patient needs. Clinicians must use their expertise and judgment to integrate patient data from monitors and physical assessments to respond appropriately.[9] This can be exhausting when health-care providers are bombarded with many alerts throughout a shift.[4,9] The Emergency Care Research Institute identified alarm fatigue and alarm-related accidents as the most severe technology hazards in health care.[5] When health-care providers develop alarm fatigue, patient safety is compromised, and adverse clinical outcomes may occur.[7,9]

PATIENT AND FAMILY IMPACT

Patients and their caregivers have significant stress when admitted to the PICU. Seeing the heartbeat on the monitors, the sounds of monitors and equipment, and the sudden sounds of monitor alarms have been identified as significant parental stressors.[10] Debelic and colleagues identified "the sudden sounds of monitor alarms" as the third-ranked stressor for parents in the PICU, ranked only behind "having a machine breathe for my child" and "not knowing how best to help my child during this crisis." Although they can be reassuring and necessary to provide care for their children, alarms can also negatively affect parental mental health as well as sleep.[11] Alarm fatigue can contribute to patients' dissatisfaction with their level of care and potential poor treatment outcomes, especially if they are unhappy with nurses' alarm response time.[11] Boston Medical Center found a strong correlation between the reduction of audible alarms and improved nursing and patient satisfaction scores. Alarms also negatively affect both patient and family rest, which can have detrimental influences on their mental and psychological health.[12] Poor sleep is also associated with the development of delirium, which is linked to increased mortality and longer hospital stays.[8]

BACKGROUND

Monitoring patients in the PICU aims to alert personnel to acute changes in a patient's condition, allowing for immediate intervention. Telemetry monitoring allows for the assessment of the heart rate and rhythm as well as conduction defects and ischemia.[13] Identification of arrhythmias promotes quick intervention that can potentially prevent cardiac arrest.[14] Cardiac arrhythmias become an emergency when hemodynamic instability develops. This hemodynamic instability can cause decreased cardiac output, which can lead to end-organ hypoperfusion.[15] Monitoring of respiratory rate can identify children with periodic apneic spells or children whose respiratory rate continues to climb despite initial interventions and may require further intervention. Continuous pulse oximetry monitoring allows for early recognition of hypoxemia while monitoring systemic oxygen saturation. A good waveform is essential for interpretation, and an inability to pick up saturations suggests potential decreased tissue perfusion.[13] Core temperature monitoring is essential in critically ill children who may require strict temperature control. This can include children with traumatic brain injuries, those who are postarrest with return of spontaneous circulation, and postoperative cardiac patients. Some patients may even require both skin temperature monitoring as well as core temperature. End-tidal CO_2 monitoring can assist with monitoring intubated patients without relying solely on blood gases. It is also helpful in nonintubated patients receiving sedating medications and requiring close monitoring of their respiratory status. Cerebral and renal Somanetics measure tissue perfusion and oxygen delivery in near-infrared spectroscopy and is helpful in assessing trends and adequacy of cardiac output. This is especially useful in postoperative cardiac patients and those children who are in shock.

Other modes of hemodynamic monitoring assist health-care providers in determining if patients have adequate tissue perfusion and initiating changes in care when perfusion is inadequate. These monitors can alert clinicians to early signs of deterioration and have great potential to help save lives. However, the monitors are notorious for generating frequent alarms, and often, these alarms are not relevant to patient safety. Bonafide and colleagues found that more than 90% of PICU alarms and more than 70% of adult intensive care alarms were not relevant to patient safety. In psychology investigations, study subjects were found to rapidly learn to ignore or respond more slowly to alarms when exposed to high false-alarm rates, leading to alarm fatigue.[16] Monitoring of pediatric patients also may occur on pediatric hospital floors, the emergency department, the operating room, and outpatient sedation services for procedures, where alarm fatigue can also develop.

When caring for children outside of the PICU, clinicians should balance the benefits of detecting potential status changes with the real risk of alarm fatigue.[17] For those patients outside of the PICU, there are very few patients for whom telemetry monitoring is indicated. These patients include those with chest pain, blunt chest trauma, acute neurological events, severe asthma exacerbation, Kawasaki disease, drug-induced dynamic measurement of the time required to reset the heart's electrical system (QTc) prolongation, syncopal event evaluation, and infants with prenatal drug exposure.[16,18] The benefit of monitoring should outweigh the risk of alarm fatigue. The Society of Hospital Medicine—Pediatric Hospital Medicine does not recommend the routine use of continuous pulse oximetry monitoring in patients unless they require supplemental oxygen.[19] Schondelmeyer and colleagues found that periodic assessment and monitoring of vital signs is appropriate for some mild or moderate conditions that require hospitalization, such as mild or moderate asthma, croup, pneumonia, and bronchiolitis. Continuous monitoring was recommended in severe diseases for

Table 1
Types of alarms encountered in the pediatric intensive care unit

Actionable Clinical Alarms	Clinical Intervention Required
Nonactionable clinical alarms	No clinical intervention required
• Invalid	• Do not reflect the actual physiologic status of the patient
• Nuisance	• Does reflect the actual physiologic status of the patient but does not require clinical intervention

respiratory infections and for patients requiring increased opiate or benzodiazepine doses. There are no national guidelines for pediatric monitors in the most common pediatric conditions. Continuous monitoring of children in the hospital outside of the PICU can identify worsening status necessitating intervention but can cause patient, parent, and health-care provider dissatisfaction if alarm fatigue ensues. Alarms can also negatively affect patients and their families by hindering sleep and increasing anxiety. Continuous monitoring may also capture regular physiologic changes, such as a brief desaturation event during the night in an otherwise healthy infant. This can cause unnecessary workup and interventions, leading to longer hospital stays.[17] Although monitors are a vital asset to patient care in the PICU, they are also infamous for producing unnecessary alarms that are not associated with an actual change in patient clinical status as is shown in **Table 1**. False alarms are those that do not reflect the patient's true status and occur regularly in the PICU. These alarms may include failure to accurately detect respiratory rate, noting cardiac arrhythmia when the patient is receiving chest physiotherapy, and low-quality pulse oximetry readings when a patient is moving.[5] Nuisance alarms, which reflect the true patient status but do not require intervention, may also occur frequently. An example would be a patient who desaturates just below the minimum acceptable pulse oximeter level for a few seconds with a return to the set parameters without intervention.[18]

Another classification of alarms is actionable versus nonactionable.[18] An actionable alarm is any alarm that alerts for a change in clinical condition that leads to clinical intervention, requires consultation with another clinician at the bedside, or alerts to a situation that should have led to intervention or consultation but was not witnessed or misinterpreted by the bedside staff. A nonactionable alarm is any alarm that does not meet actionable alarm standards. These may be caused by motion artifacts, equipment/technical alarms, and alarms that represent a change in patient condition but do not require intervention or consultation. When health-care providers are exposed to many nonactionable alarms, they are less likely to respond promptly to future actionable alarms.[16]

DISCUSSION

PICU nurses are lauded for their attention to detail and specialized care of critically ill children but even they can fall victim to alarm fatigue as is expressed in **Fig. 1**. What can lessen this phenomenon to protect these vulnerable patients better? Karnik and colleagues developed a framework to minimize alarm fatigue.[18] The following interventions were suggested.

- Monitoring only those patients that are at significant risk of a life-threatening event
- Reducing invalid (artifact) alarms
- Reducing nuisance (valid but nonactionable) alarms
- Improving alarm notification for the remaining actionable alarms

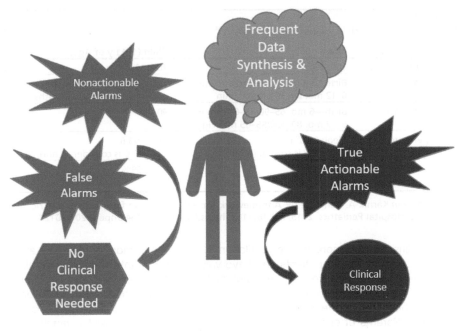

Fig. 1. Nursing assessment of clinical alarms.

The primary goal of electrocardiographic monitoring is to detect arrhythmia. Respiratory compromise often precedes cardiac center in children except those with congenital heart disease. Early recognition and treatment of children with circulatory insufficiency or shock are crucial to improving their survival.[20] This early recognition relies on monitors and appropriate alarms to alert staff to changes in the patient's condition, necessitating acute intervention. Once a child improves, providers should regularly evaluate the necessity of continuous monitors in their care.

Another intervention to reduce alarm fatigue is to reduce invalid (artifact) alarms. Invalid alarms occur when there is poor or inadequate contact between the patient's skin and the electrodes and are often caused either by the electrode's sensor drying out or by the patient movement. When monitoring is indicated in patients, even when awake and active, meticulous skin care and changing electrodes every 24 hours can help decrease these alarms.

Reducing nuisance alarms is another intervention suggested to decrease alarm fatigue. Nuisance alarms often occur when alarm thresholds are set at levels in which intervention is not warranted or when the patient alarms for an appropriate threshold but is only briefly out of range and requires no intervention. One solution to these alarms is to set alarm thresholds at appropriate ranges for the age of the child being monitored. Normal vital sign ranges for infants and children can be seen in **Table 2**. For example, the 1st and 99th percentile for age for heart rate and respiratory rate could be the initial alarm threshold set. These thresholds can then be adjusted for the needs of each individual patient to minimize the occurrence of nonactionable alarms.[18] Patients in the PICU may not have normal vital signs due to either their critical illness or underlying disease process. When setting the initial alarm thresholds, the patient's history and condition should be considered.[5] For example, a child with complex congenital heart disease who has single ventricle physiology will have different pulse oximetry settings than the previously healthy patient with

Table 2
Normal infant and child vital sign parameters[23,24]

	Infant	Child (1–11 y of Age)
Heart rate (bpm)	100–160	70–120
Respiratory rate	Birth to 6 mo: 30–60 breaths/min 6–12 mo: 24–30 breaths/min	1–5 y of age: 20–30 breaths/min 6–11 y of age: 12–20 breaths/min
Blood pressure	Birth—6 mo: 65–90/45–65 mm Hg 6–12 mo: 80–100/55–65 mm Hg	90–110/55–75 mm Hg
Temperature	Ideal: 98.6⁰ F 97.4–99.6 is considered normal	Ideal: 98.6 97.4–99.6 is considered normal
Oxygenation via pulse oximetry	90%–100%	97%–99%

Adapted from Karnik A, Bonafide CP. A framework for reducing alarm fatigue on pediatric inpatient units. Hospital Pediatrics. 2015;5(3):160-163. https://doi.org/10.1542/hpeds.2014-0123.

bronchiolitis requiring noninvasive ventilation. Nurses spend most of their time at the bedside caring for these patients and have valuable insight into whether their alarm parameters are appropriately set. Although institutional policies vary, allowing nurses to adjust monitor alarm parameters within a safe margin without a physician order may be beneficial if the physician and care team is notified and aware of the change.[18] Parents of chronically critically ill children can also assist in establishing appropriate alarm limits for their child.[5] When families participate in patient care and decision-making as well as information sharing, this may also help manage alarm fatigue.[5]

Another step to decrease alarm fatigue is to institute a delay in the time interval before an alarm sounds. The goal would be to reduce recurrent alarms for short, self-limited breaches of the alarm thresholds. A pulse oximetry called SatSeconds (Nellcor device, Medtronic Minneapolis, MN, USA) can account for both the depth and the duration of a desaturation event and will immediately alarm for a major desaturation event but will delay an alarm for a less significant drop in oxygenation.[18]

The final suggested action by Karnik and colleagues was to improve alarm recognition and notification for actionable alarms. Alarms are only valuable for clinicians if observed and their acuity is acknowledged. Suggestions to overcome these barriers are secondary notification systems and monitor watchers. Secondary notification systems can alert a nurse to an alarm via a pager or phone system. The alert can be escalated to the charge nurses or another designated clinician if the bedside nurse does not respond. "Monitor watchers" are personnel hired to continuously view and monitor patients from a central station who then notify staff as needed of alarms requiring immediate attention.[18]

The National Patient Safety Goals (NPSG) effective for January 2023 include reducing patient harm associated with clinical alarm systems and can be seen in **Box 1**. The primary goal aims to improve the safety of clinical alarm systems. The NPSG recognizes that clinical alarm systems are meant to alert clinicians to possible changes in patient status that require attention; however, if these alarms are not adequately managed, they can negatively influence patient safety. Alarm fatigue is a complex issue with multiple causes, some of which include too many alarms (these can desensitize staff and cause them to ignore alarms, essential or not), inappropriate alarm settings, and inadequate default alarm settings. The NPSG (2023) encourages hospital leaders to establish alarm system safety as a hospital priority.[21] The ultimate goal of hospitals is to provide care in the safest way possible. One way patient safety

---

Box 1
Element(s) of performance for NPSG.06.01.01

1. Leaders establish alarm system safety as a hospital priority.

2. Identify the most important alarm signals to manage based on the following:
   - Input from the medical staff and clinical departments
   - Risk to patients if the alarm signal is not attended to or if it malfunctions
   - Whether specific alarm signals are needed or unnecessarily contribute to alarm noise and alarm fatigue
   - Potential for patient harm based on internal incident history
   - Published best practices and guidelines

3. Establish policies and procedures for managing the alarms identified in EP 2 above that, at a minimum, address the following:
   - Clinically appropriate settings for alarm signals
   - When alarm signals can be disabled
   - When alarm parameters can be changed
   - Who in the organization has the authority to set alarm parameters
   - Who in the organization has the authority to change alarm parameters
   - Who in the organization can set alarm parameters to "off"
   - Monitoring and responding to alarm signals
   - Checking individual alarm signals for accurate settings, proper operation, and detectability

4. Educate staff and licensed independent practitioners about the purpose and proper operation of alarm systems for which they are responsible.

---

can be negatively affected is by alarm fatigue. Hospitals and PICUs can combat alarm fatigue by taking several steps, including setting appropriate alarm limits, only monitoring essential physiologic parameters, and having a monitor tech assist with identifying those alarms that require immediate attention.

RECOMMENDATIONS

- Collaborate with the care team to customize parameters to the patient and set alarm defaults to ± 10% of patients' baseline
- Pause alarms when performing care that creates nonactionable alarms
- Change electrocardiography (ECG) electrodes daily and place leads correctly with proper skin preparation
- Change pulse oximeter sensors as needed and ensure skin integrity under the probe
- Discontinue monitoring devices as soon as no longer clinically necessary

SUMMARY

The advent of monitors in modern medicine has allowed clinicians to recognize and intervene early in changing patient conditions and move from a reactionary mode of patient care to one that can potentially prevent clinical decompensation. Despite these positive attributes, alarms can create alarm fatigue, which remains one of the most significant safety concerns in patient care today. Research has shown that patients and caregivers can be exposed to up to 180 alarms in a 12-hour shift in the intensive care unit.[22–24] These alarms can include monitor alarms, ventilator alarms, and intravenous (IV) pump alarms. Without intervention, staff can be desensitized to these alarms, leading to increased response times and delayed intervention times. Jubic stated, "Identifying causes for alarm fatigue, managing alarm fatigue, and determining the impact of alarm fatigue on nurses can assist in the prevention of adverse clinical events and ensure prompt assessment of a patient's condition." Nurses should use age-specific and patient-specific parameters and discuss the need for monitoring with the entire care team as needed. As Jubic notes, by preventing alarm fatigue, a trusting and therapeutic care environment is created that supports the well-being of critically ill pediatric patients.[5] This environment may also positively influence the family-centered experience by providing families with the comfort that their child's alarms will be quickly attended to. Nurses should remain empowered to be an active part of the patient care team and ensure that the technology will contribute to improved patient outcomes.

CLINICS CARE POINTS

- Health-care workers are exposed to hundreds of alarms in a standard intensive care unit shift.
- Studies have shown that most alarms in the PICU (90%) are false or nonactionable.
- Exposure to so many nonactionable alarms causes health-care provider desensitization to future alarms.
- Alarm desensitization can lead to prolonged time to recognize and respond to a change in a patient's condition.
- Alarm fatigue is the most significant technology concern in health care.
- Health-care teams need to take steps to mitigate the number of alarms nurses are exposed to in a shift.

CONFLICTS OF INTEREST

Both authors have no conflicts of interest to disclose.

REFERENCES

1. Vincent JL. Critical Care – where have we been, and where are we going? Crit Care 2013;17.
2. Kelly FE, Fong K, Hirsch N, et al. Intensive care medicine is 60 years old: the history and future of the intensive care unit. Clin Med 2014;14(4):376–9.
3. Hannibal GB. It started with Einthoven: the history of the ECG and cardiac monitoring. AACN Adv Crit Care 2011;22(1):93–6.
4. Drew FA. Patient monitors in critical care: lessons for improvement, In: Henriksen K, Battles JB, Keyes MA, et al. Approaches to patient safety: new directions and alternative approaches, vol. 3, 2008, Agency for Healthcare Research and Quality; Rockville (MD), Performance and tools. AHRQ Publication No. 08-0034-3. Available at: https://www.ncbi.nlm.nih.gov/books/NBK43684/.
5. Jubic K. Strategies for managing alarm fatigue in the PICU setting. Pediatr Nurs 2017;43(5).
6. Suleman Z, Manning JC, Evans C. Parents' and carers' experiences of transitions and aftercare following a child discharge from a pediatric intensive care unit to an inpatient ward setting: a qualitative systematic review protocol. JBI Database of Systematic Reviews and Implementation Reports 2016;14(1):89–98.
7. Turmell JW, Coke L, Catinella R, et al. Alarm fatigue: use of an evidence-based alarm management strategy. J Nurs Care Qual 2017;32(1):47–54.

8. PICU Alarm Fatigue - Projects - UR Health Lab - University of Rochester Medical Center. Available at: www.urmc.rochester.edu. https://www.urmc.rochester.edu/health-lab/projects/picu-alarm-fatigue.aspx. Accessed January 27, 2023.

9. Ruskin KJ, Hueske-Kraus D. Alarm fatigue: impacts on patient safety. Curr Opin Anaesthesiol 2015;28(6):685–90.

10. Upadhyay V, Parashar Y. A study of parental stressors, financial issues as stress factor, and the coping Strategies in the PICU. Indian J Pediatr 2022. https://doi.org/10.1007/s12098-021-04003-0.

11. What Is Alarm Fatigue? Tips for Prevention. Maryville Online. Published January 4, 2022. Available at: https://online.maryville.edu/blog/what-is-alarm-fatigue/#:~:text=Since%20alarm%20fatigue%20also%20impacts%20nurses%E2%80%99. Accessed January 27, 2023.

12. Burdick KJ, Callahan CJ. Sleeping soundlessly in the intensive care unit. Multimodal Technol Interact 2020;4(1):6.

13. University of Iowa Stead Family Children's Hospital. Monitoring Devices: PICU Handbook. Available at: Monitoring Devices: PICU Handbook | University of Iowa Stead Family Children's Hospital (uihc.org). Accessed January 26, 2023.

14. Mick NW, Williams RJ. Pediatric cardiac arrest resuscitation. Emerg Med Clin N Am 2020;38:819–39.

15. Watnick, C. and Otillio, J. K. (2015). Assessing and managing pediatric cardiac rhythm disturbances. Journal of Emergency Medical Services, published January 26, 2015. Available at: Assessing and Managing Pediatric Cardiac Rhythm Disturbances - JEMS: EMS, Emergency Medical Services - Training, Paramedic, EMT NewsF. Accessed January 30, 2023.

16. Bonafide C, Lin R, Zander M, et al. Association between exposure to nonactionable physiologic monitor alarms and response time in a children's hospital. Hosp Med 2015;10(6):345–51.

17. Schondelmeyer A, Dewan ML, Brady PW, et al. Cardiorespiratory and pulse oximetry monitoring in hospitalized children: a Delphi process. Pediatrics 2020; 146(2). https://doi.org/10.1542/peds.2019-3336.

18. Karnik A, Bonafide CP. A framework for reducing alarm fatigue on pediatric inpatient units. Hosp Pediatr 2015;5(3):160–3.

19. Society of Hospital Medicine – Pediatric Hospital Medicine. Choosing Wisely. Available at: https://choosingwisely.org. Accessed January 18, 2023.

20. Singh Y, Villascusa JU, da Cruz EM, et al. Recommendations for hemodynamic monitoring for critically ill children – expert consensus statement issued by the cardiovascular dynamics section of the European Society of Paediatric and Neonatal Intensive Care (ESPNIC). Crit Care 2020;24:62.

21. The Joint Commission (2022). National patient safety goals effective January 2023 for the hospital program. Available at: National Patient Safety Goals | The Joint Commission.

22. Lewis, CL, Oster, CA. Research outcomes of implementing CEASE: An innovative, nurse-driven, evidence-based, patient-customized monitoring bundle to decrease alarm fatigue in the intensive care unit/step-down unit. Dimensions of Critical Care Nursing. 2019;34(3):160-173.

23. Pediatric Vital Signs: A Guide for Nurses. Ohio University. Published April 5, 2021. Available at: https://onlinemasters.ohio.edu/blog/pediatric-vital-signs/#:~:text="' Normal%20vital%20signs%20for%20children%20are%20as%20follows%3A.

24. PEARS Vital signs in children. American Academy of Pediatrics. 9e73fdf903867 a823559e2d50e67a50c.jpg (736×1185) (pinimg.com). Accessed January 30, 2023.

Moving?

Make sure your subscription moves with you!

To notify us of your new address, find your **Clinics Account Number** (located on your mailing label above your name), and contact customer service at:

Email: journalscustomerservice-usa@elsevier.com

800-654-2452 (subscribers in the U.S. & Canada)
314-447-8871 (subscribers outside of the U.S. & Canada)

Fax number: 314-447-8029

**Elsevier Health Sciences Division
Subscription Customer Service
3251 Riverport Lane
Maryland Heights, MO 63043**

*To ensure uninterrupted delivery of your subscription, please notify us at least 4 weeks in advance of move.